Tobacco
and
Oral Health

TEXT AND COLOR ATLAS

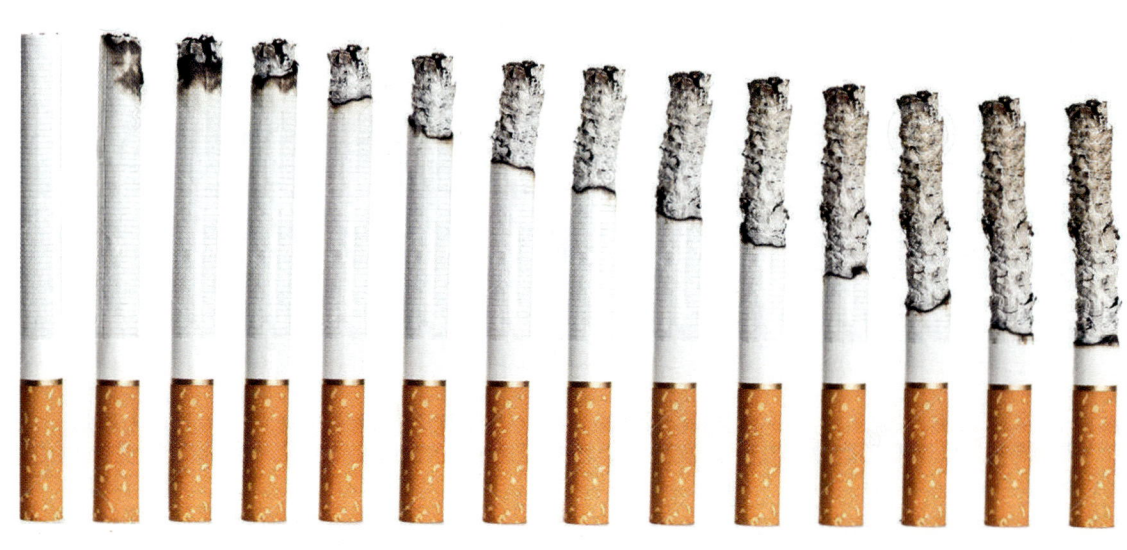

Tobacco
and
Oral Health

TEXT AND COLOR ATLAS

Tanushree Keswani BDS MDS

School of Dental Sciences, Sharda University
Oral Medicine and Radiology
Subharti Dental College and Hospital
Swami Vivekanand Subharti University
Meerut, Uttar Pradesh

Assisted by

Sreenivasan Venkatraman

Professor and Head
Department of Oral Medicine and Radiology
Saraswati-Dhanwantri Dental College and Hospital
Parbhani, Maharashtra

Ravi Prakash SM MDS

Professor and Head
Department of Oral Medicine and Radiology
Subharti Dental College and Hospital
Meerut, Uttar Pradesh

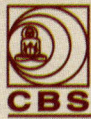

CBS

CBS Publishers & Distributors Pvt Ltd

New Delhi • Bengaluru • Chennai • Kochi • Kolkata • Mumbai
Hyderabad • Nagpur • Patna • Pune • Vijayawada

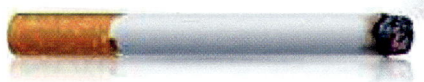

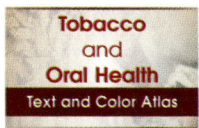

ISBN: 978-81-239-2859-3

First Edition: 2016

Published by Satish Kumar Jain and produced by Varun Jain for

CBS Publishers & Distributors Pvt Ltd

4819/XI Prahlad Street, 24 Ansari Road, Daryaganj, New Delhi 110 002, India.
Ph: 23289259, 23266861, 23266867   Website: www.cbspd.com
Fax: 011-23243014   e-mail: delhi@cbspd.com; cbspubs@airtelmail.in.
Corporate Office: 204 FIE, Industrial Area, Patparganj, Delhi 110 092
Ph: 4934 4934   Fax: 4934 4935   e-mail: publishing@cbspd.com; publicity@cbspd.com

Branches

- **Bengaluru:** Seema House 2975, 17th Cross, K.R. Road,
  Banasankari 2nd Stage, Bengaluru 560 070, Karnataka
  Ph: +91-80-26771678/79   Fax: +91-80-26771680   e-mail: bangalore@cbspd.com
- **Chennai:** 7, Subbaraya Street, Shenoy Nagar, Chennai 600 030, Tamil Nadu
  Ph: +91-44-26680620, 26681266   Fax: +91-44-42032115   e-mail: chennai@cbspd.com
- **Kochi:** Ashana House, No. 39/1904, AM Thomas Road, Valanjambalam, Ernakulam 682 018, Kochi, Kerala
  Ph: +91-484-4059061-65   Fax: +91-484-4059065   e-mail: kochi@cbspd.com
- **Kolkata:** 6/B, Ground Floor, Rameswar Shaw Road, Kolkata-700 014, West Bengal
  Ph: +91-33-22891126, 22891127, 22891128   e-mail: kolkata@cbspd.com
- **Mumbai:** 83-C, Dr E Moses Road, Worli, Mumbai-400018, Maharashtra
  Ph: +91-22-24902340/41   Fax: +91-22-24902342   e-mail: mumbai@cbspd.com

Representatives

- **Hyderabad** 0-9885175004   • **Nagpur**   0-9021734563   • **Patna** 0-9334159340
- **Pune**   0-9623451994   • **Vijayawada** 0-9000660880

Printed at: Magic International Pvt. Ltd., Greater Noida

to

---

my beloved Master

my amorous grandmother
Mrs Lajwanti Khemchandani

my godly parents
Asha Keswani and MK Keswani

my doting siblings
Richa and Raman Keswani

Contributors

Tanushree Keswani
School of Dental Sciences, Sharda University
Oral Medicine and Radiology
Subharti Dental College and Hospital
Swami Vivekanand Subharti University
Meerut, UP

Nagaraju K
Reader, Department of Oral Medicine and Radiology
Subharti Dental College, Meerut, UP

Swati Goel
Senior Lecturer, Department of
Oral Medicine and Radiology
Subharti Dental College, Meerut, UP

Swati Gupta
Postgraduate Student
Department of Oral Medicine and Radiology
Subharti Dental College, Meerut, UP

Sangeeta Malik
Reader, Department of Oral Medicine and Radiology
Subharti Dental College
Meerut, UP

Sumit Goel
Reader, Department of Oral Medicine and Radiology
Subharti Dental College
Meerut, UP

Renuka J Bathi
Professor, Department of Oral Medicine and Radiology
Jodhpur Dental College
Rajasthan

Tarun Sharma
Assistant Professor
Seema Dental College
Rishikesh

Foreword

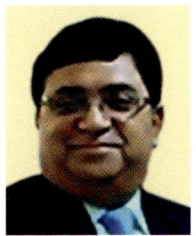

Tobacco has a distinct pattern in India. Dental care professionals need to come together to contribute and assist their patients in a more emphatic manner.

I congratulate the authors in their effort to compile such a comprehensive collection of facts and photographs. The information provided is interesting and tactfully presented. This novel approach would not only allow it to be integrated into dental curriculum but also augment the introduction of applied teaching methodology into tobacco control. The authors have really amazed me with their sheer effort to compile such glimpses into the habit, rooted in our country. This effort shall surely make an everlasting imprint onto the mind of its readers. The book is seeking to engage the students in a positive manner to understand the nuances of tobacco use in our country, through its illustrations.

I am sure this publication will be a great boon to undergraduate and postgraduate dental and medical students and provide them a better lens to view the same old problem.

I am pleased to be asked by the authors to write the Foreword to the book *Tobacco and Oral Health* TEXT AND COLOR ATLAS. I wish them success in their endeavor.

Maheshverma

Mahesh Verma
Director-Principal
Maulana Azad Institute of Dental Sciences
New Delhi

Foreword

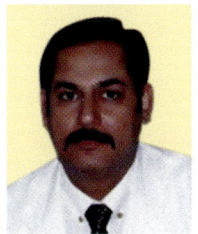

I feel gratified and proud to be asked by my student to proffer a foreword to this book *Tobacco and Oral Health* TEXT AND COLOR ATLAS which is the outcome of hard work and collective effort by the authors and other eminent and dedicated academicians.

Since every clinician and particularly our budding doctors are always in a quest to learn and quench their thirst for pathology and physiology, this book will act like a guiding light for students and learners to distinguish between normal and abnormal findings.

There is a relatively low awareness about the oro-mucosal lesions amongst a large section of health professionals. A number of clinical photographs compiled in the ATLAS will help them be acquainted with this territory and thus be enlightened. The book also showcases a wide variety of tobacco forms and related oral mucosal lesions that may be seen and collected only after many years of experience and prodigious practice.

I have no doubt that this book will immensely benefit both the students and the clinicians in diagnosing various complex conditions and providing quality oro-dental care to the patients.

Nikhil Srivastava
Professor and Head
Pedodontics and Preventive Dentistry
Principal, Subharti Dental College and Hospital
Dean, Faculty of Dental Sciences
Swami Vivekanand Subharti University
Meerut (INDIA)

Preface

In the world of commercial speech, tobacco advertising
bears the earmarks of an endangered species

Tobacco, delicious father of abiding friendships and fertile reveries.
—Luis B: Little tube of mighty pow'r

Tobacco is the second major cause of death worldwide, and responsible for about 5 million deaths annually. This figure is expected to rise to about 8.4 million by the year 2020, with 70% of those deaths occurring in the developing countries. The smoking prevalence males (% of adults) in India was 26.25 in 2009, according to a World Bank report, published in 2010. It is the need of the hour to reduce the use of tobacco to decrease the associated morbidity and mortality.

As dentists, we often come across patients with tobacco habits, and are in a stronger position compared to other medical practitioners to identify oral changes in these patients and counsel the patients regarding the adverse effects of tobacco. The use of smokeless tobacco is associated with a spectrum of oral cavity lesions, including leukoplakia, speckled leukoplakia, erythroplakia, tobacco-associated keratosis, carcinoma *in situ* (CIS), verrucous carcinoma, and invasive squamous cell carcinoma (SCC). It can cause smokeless tobacco-induced keratosis, gingival inflammation, periodontal inflammation, alveolar bone damage, dental caries, and tooth abrasion.

The volume is compiled with a view to investigate the types of tobacco habits in various parts of India. Two sections of the book showcase different forms of tobacco prevalent in India. The first section collates tobacco forms that have been collected from patients and the second section compiles a collection of tobacco forms derived from the published literature.

Along with showcasing the normal variants of oral mucosa, it shows a wide variety of oral lesions and briefs on how to properly correlate all available findings in interpreting the lesions. To do justice to the significance of early signs of prognostically serious diseases and to emphasize the responsibility of the dentist as the first examiner, emphasis is given to malignant tumors of the oral cavity together with their precursors. It brings to light the importance of tobacco cessation clinics and the profound impact it has on bringing about the most important change in lives of tobacco users.

The assorted clinical photographs are garnered according to the anatomical sites of oral mucosa, thereby emphasizing both common and uncommon sites of occurrence of each of these lesions.

Tanushree Keswani

Acknowledgments

I thank and acknowledge the members of the institution, Subharti Dental College, especially the faculty of Department of Oral Medicine and Radiology, where the concept of this work was born and accomplished. I express gratitude to Dr Nikhil Srivastava, Principal, Subharti Dental College, for providing adequate facilities and guidance. I am indebted to my mentor, Dr V Sreenivasan, without whom this book would have never seen light of the day.

Most importantly, all the patients, who allowed themselves to be photographed and be incorporated this volume.

I feel indebted to Dr Jagadeesh HG, Principal, School of Dental Sciences, Sharda University, and Dr Renuka J Bathi for their prodigious backing and affection for me.

No amount of words can express my gratefulness towards my saintly teachers Natarajan Sir and Kalyani madam, who have always been my guiding light in all respects.

I will be ever obligated to Dr Tarun Sharma, Assistant Professor, Seema Dental College, Rishikesh, for his selfless advice and support.

I hold deep affection and respect for my maternal uncle and aunt, Vijay Khemchandani and Kiran Makhija, respectively, for being my pillars of strength since my childhood.

I am thankful to my teachers Dr Pooja Kabra and Dr Swati Sharma, Readers, School of Dental Sciences, Sharda University.

Tanushree Keswani

Contents

Cigarette, a fire at one end, a fool at the other, and a bit of tobacco in between

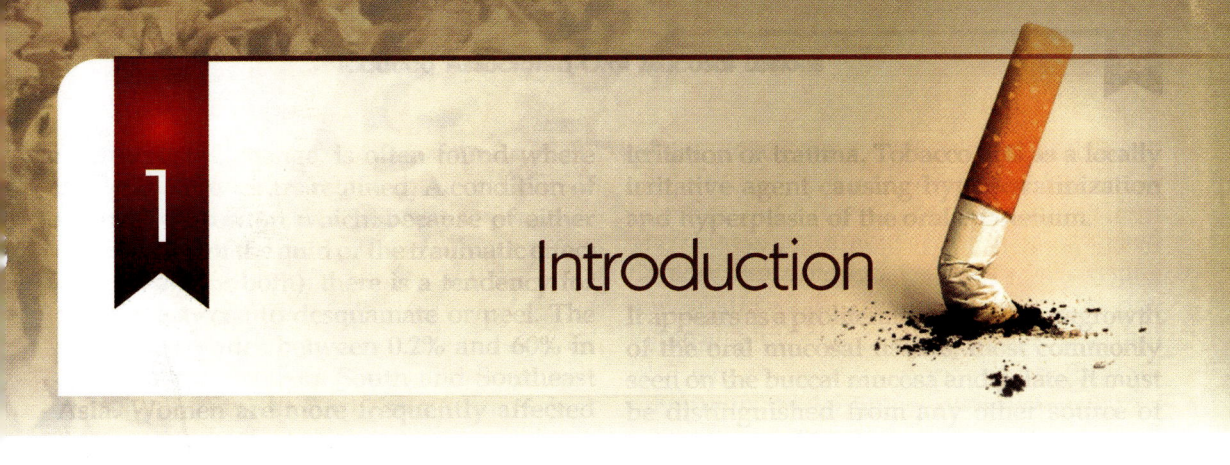

Introduction

Tobacco—a transitory pleasure; that invites a future of disease, death and horror.

Tobacco use has encompassed our lives in all spheres—social, occupational, economic and political. Currently 5.1 million people die every year globally from tobacco use, of which 1.2 million are from the South-East Asian (SEA) region alone. In India, as in most low income countries, death in middle age is increasing in relative importance due to an increase in smoking related deaths. The disease burden, health care costs as well as other fiscal losses resulting from premature deaths attributable to tobacco consumption will rapidly increase. Earlier WHO estimates suggest that deaths and disability adjusted life years (DALYs) attributable to tobacco use in India will increase from 1,29,000 deaths and 1719 DALYs in 1990 to over 1.5 million deaths and 24,024 DALYs by 2002.

Tobacco use causes a wide range of major diseases which impact nearly every organ of the body. Tobacco-related illnesses such as cancer and cardiovascular and respiratory diseases are already major problems in most countries. There are many dangerous health risks that tobacco use poses such as coronary artery disease, sudden cardiac death, cardiac arrhythmias, cerebrovascular accidents, thromboangiitis obliterans, abdominal aortic aneurysms, renal artery stenosis and respiratory diseases like pneumonia, bronchitis and other acute respiratory infections. Exposure to second-hand tobacco smoke has also been conclusively shown to cause lung cancer. Evidence to support that there is an increased frequency of chromosomal damage among those chewing tobacco is documented.

Oral and pharyngeal cancers, caused due to direct contact with carcinogens in smokeless tobacco products and tobacco smoke, have a high incidence in the SEA region even among women, due to the prevalence of smokeless tobacco use in various forms. Despite advances in treatment and reconstructive surgery, there has been no improvement in oral cancer prognosis for over four decades. It would seem that the key to better quality and length of survival is more effective detection of disease at a premalignant stage or when the invasive lesion is small. Today the future is relatively optimistic for patients whose disease is identified early. These mucosal changes caused due to smoke and smokeless tobacco may range from trivial chemical burn, lichenoid reaction, snuff dipper's lesion, nicotinic stomatitis, tobacco pouch keratosis; to potentially malignant disorders like leukoplakia, erythroplakia, oral submucous fibrosis. Such lesions if not diagnosed in time can undergo malignant transformation. According to a re-evaluation in 2004 by the International Agency for Research of Cancer both betel quid and areca nut have been considered to be Group 1 or 'carcinogenic to humans' (Jacob et al., 2004; Lee et al., 2005). The concept of precancerous lesions proceeding into oral cancer has long been accepted (Gupta et al., 1989; Yen et al., 2007).

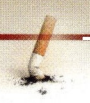

According to a workshop co-ordinated by WHO in May 2005 at London the use of the term 'potentially malignant disorders' was recommended. The usage of this terminology conveys that not all lesions and conditions described under this term may transform to cancer, instead there is a family of morphological alterations amongst which some may have an increased potential for malignant transformation (Warnakulasuriya et al., 2007; Chong et al., 2011).

Chewing, smoking and consumption of alcoholic beverages have become common social habits in India. According to national cross sectional household survey, 2003; sixteen per cent of the study population (29.3% men and 2.3% women) smoked tobacco; 20% of the study population (28.1% men and 12.0% women) chewed tobacco/pan masala; and 30% of the study population (46.5% men and 13.8% women) either smoked or chewed tobacco. Since the consumption of tobacco and its forms is on a rise in our country, so are the everincreasing adverse effects too. It is not necessary that a student or a clinician, in his/her practical tenure may come across all the diverse alterations and lesions caused due to tobacco usage.

Thus, this color atlas displays an exorbitant number and types of tobacco related lesions with emphasis on the cause, diagnosis and treatment of these very lesions. Since it is of utmost importance to distinguish normal variants from the abnormal ones, a section on the former has also been put forth.

Forms of Tobacco

An evil with many faces

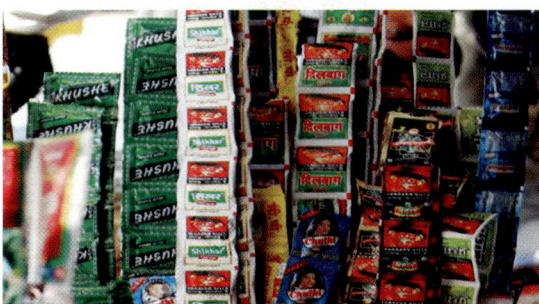 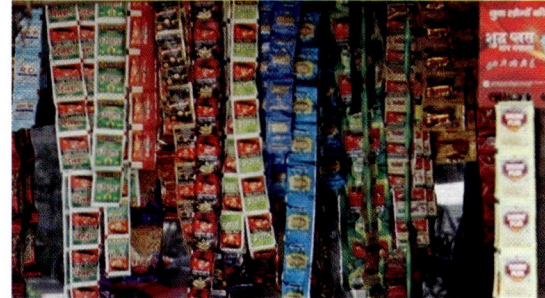

Fig. 2.1: Easy availability of tobacco and its products.

> The true face of tobacco consumption is disease, death and horror—not the glamour and sophistication the pushers in the tobacco industry try to portray.
> —*David Byrne*

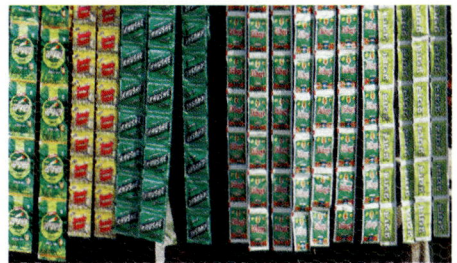

A collection of different kinds of brands of tobacco consumed by the population of Northern India is portrayed for a better understanding of these forms. In Northern India, it was found that the most popular forms of tobacco use, as smoke was bidi, cigarette and hookah; and; as smokeless forms were gutkha and dried tobacco. Several social, environmental and cultural factors were associated with tobacco consumption initiation. Easy accessibility to tobacco products and advertising, parental and sibling smoking, peer pressure and the perceived benefits of tobacco such as beliefs about mood control and positive image of smoking contributed to youth smoking.

SMOKING FORMS

In a majority of researches conducted in India, smoke forms have predominated the tobacco forms consumed by the population. This form seems to rule the masses due to its low cost and ease of use.

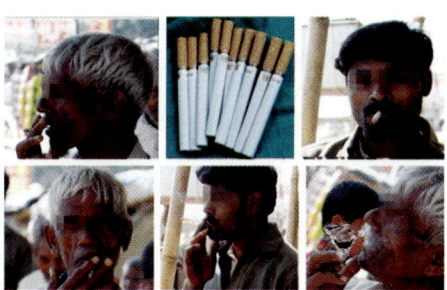

Bidis

In bidis, the most popular brand used was *Kalpana bidi*, which was due to a convenient and relatively sophisticated packaging. Other brands in use were *502 Pataka bidi*.

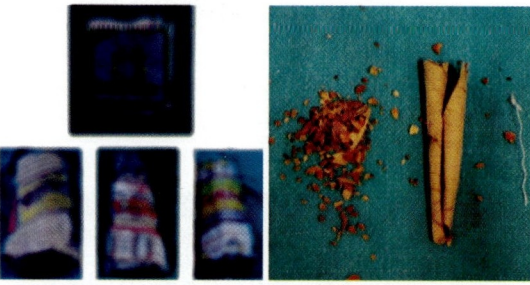

Fig. 2.2: Various kinds of brands of bidi used by the population of Northern India, Uttar Pradesh. A bidi preparation comprising of a rectangular piece of the temburni leaf with grated tobacco, rolled and secured with a thread.

In this region, bidis (*pronounced bee-dee*) are commonly used, that consist of a small amount of tobacco, hand-wrapped in dried temburni leaf and tied with string. Despite their small size, their tar and carbon monoxide deliveries can be higher than manufactured cigarettes because of the need to puff harder to keep bidis lit.

Cigarettes

Manufactured cigarettes consist of shredded orre constituted tobacco processed with hundreds of chemicals. Often with a filter, they are manufactured by a machine, and are, the predominant form of tobacco used worldwide.

Among cigarettes, the eminent forms were *Wills* (*Classic, Light* and *Navy Cut* varieties) *and Gold Flake*. Products labeled as "light" cigarettes may have been viewed by consumers as less addictive or toxic than full-flavor varieties. Ventilation holes in the filters of "light" cigarettes were designed to provide the impression that the smoker is experiencing a reduction in the exposure to tobacco smoke and its constituents. However, it has become apparent that existing reduced harm tobacco

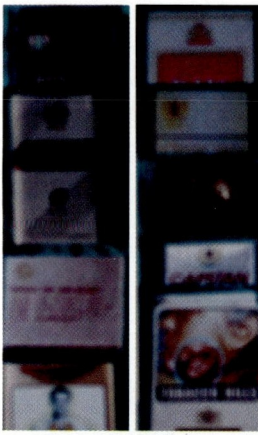

Fig. 2.3: Various kinds of cigarette brands used by the population of Northern India, Uttar Pradesh.

products, such as brands formerly marketed as "light", present no obvious reduction in harm compared with regular, full flavor products. Moreover, it is now clear that smokers compensate for increased filter ventilation in "light" cigarettes by modifying their puffing behavior. Modifications include stronger puffing (i.e. larger and more frequent) that potentially results in higher nicotine, tar, and carbon monoxide extraction. Furthermore, it has been suggested that changes in smoking behavior (e.g. stronger puffs) contribute to increases in carcinogen exposure (per cigarette), as well as changes in the concentrations of other smoke constituents.

Hookah

Hookah/water pipe was especially common among the rural population, as being a family tradition followed and passed on by the ancestors. The increasing trend of water pipe smoking can be attributed to several misconceptions. These include the popular beliefs that the nicotine content in water pipes is lower as compared to cigarettes and that the water used in this form of tobacco intake filters out all the hazardous chemicals such as carbon monoxide, nicotine and tar. These common misconceptions lead the public to believe that water pipe smoking is not a significant health hazard. Research however has proved otherwise, suggesting three additional risks of water pipe smoking over cigarette smoking. First of all water pipe is smoked over coal adding additional harmful toxins to the smoke. Secondly, a water pipe smoker's inhales up to 200 times more smoke in a single session as compared to cigarette smokers. It is linked to high rates of second-hand smoking due to its high social acceptance. Water pipe smoking, just as cigarette smoking, has been associated with increased rates of pulmonary, gastrointestinal, cardiovascular and hematological disease. A possible involvement of the tobacco industry is also suggested by researchers. A recent study done in Pakistan showed that curiosity followed by pleasure seeking and boredom were the most important factors in starting water pipe smoking. The majority of these participants thought of cigarette smoking as being more harmful as compared to water pipe smoking. Another study in Syria showed that water pipe and cigarette smoking are common among university students, with regular usage with cigarette smoking and occasional water pipe smoking.

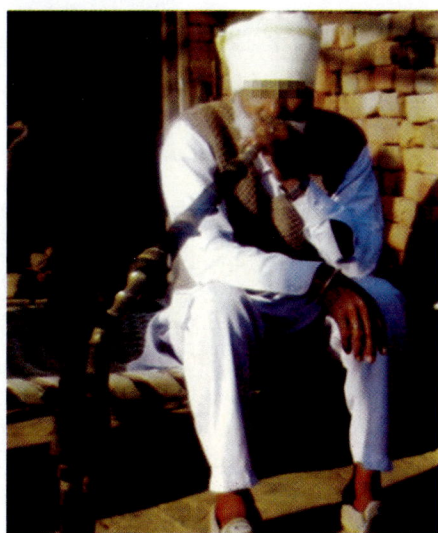

Fig. 2.4: Water pipe/hookah used more commonly by the rural population of Northern India.

Smokeless Forms

Pan masala, or betel quid consists of tobacco, areca nuts and slaked lime wrapped in a betel leaf. They can also contain other sweetening and flavouring agents.

Supari

Sweety supari was a form of branded areca nut, that was commonly and routinely consumed by female and child population, in this region.

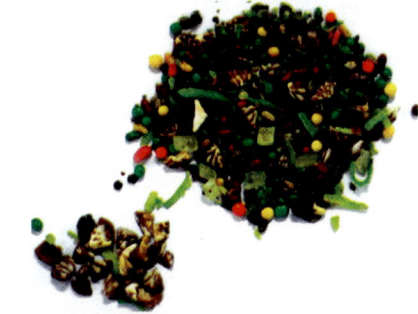

Fig. 2.5: Locally available areca nut mixed with saunf, elaichi and sugar coated balls.

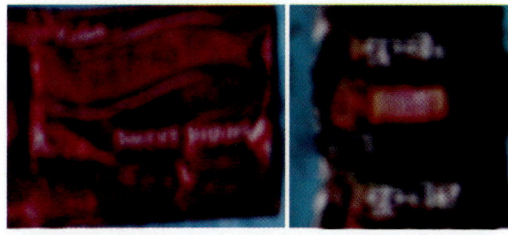

Fig. 2.6: Various kinds of chewable forms of sliced areca nut/supari.

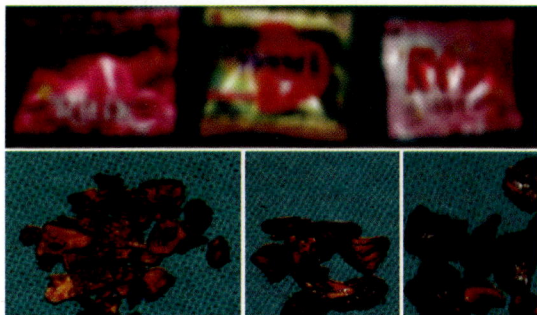

Fig. 2.7: Different varieties of flavored supari available in some parts of South India. Different slice/grain sizes and texture of brands are seen across the country.

Dried Tobacco

In the chewable, plain tobacco variety, the most preferred brand was *Kuber* and *Nevla*.

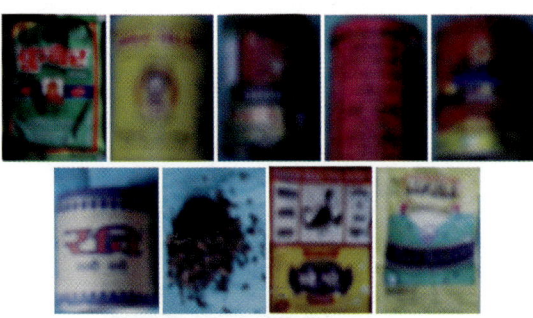

Fig. 2.8: Different types of dried tobacco available in Northern India, Uttar Pradesh.

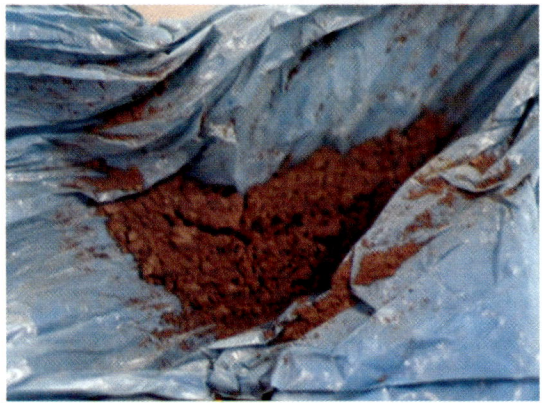

Fig. 2.9: Finely ground tobacco mixed with ash and consumed by the rural population of Northern India.

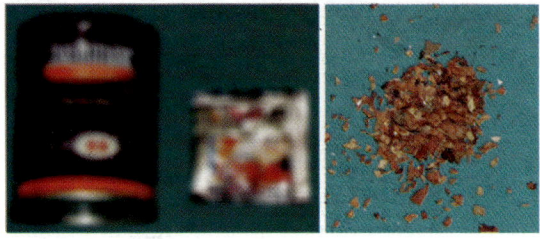

Fig. 2.10: Two most commonly used forms of plain tobacco in some parts of the country.

Gutkha

Among gutkha chewers, the popular brands were *Dabang* and *Pradhan*.

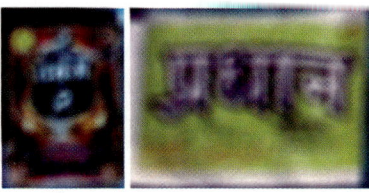

Fig. 2.11: Varieties of gutkha seen in Northern India.

Pan Masala

Dilbaag and *Rajnigandha pan masala* was especially popular among the youth. This appeared to be related to the pervasiveness of advertising and youth's belief that it is more exclusive, and of better quality, an image intensively promoted by the tobacco company.

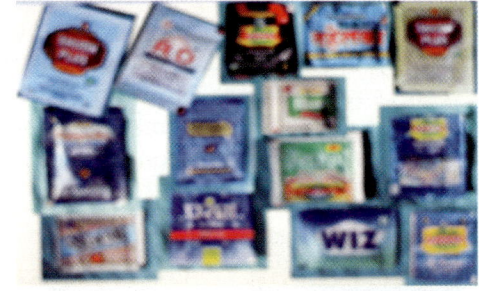

Fig. 2.12: Variable varieties of pan masala consumed by people of Northern India.

Khaini

People who consumed *khaini* (tobacco mixed with slaked lime) used the locally available pouches or bottled variety of tobacco and slaked lime. The ones who preferred pre-mixed varieties of khaini used *Chaini Khaini* and *Safal,* colloquially known as the filtered variety.

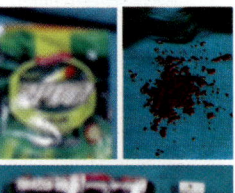

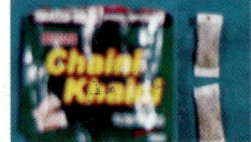

Fig. 2.13: A khaini preparation, in unfiltered and filtered forms.

Tobacco and Slaked Lime Preparation

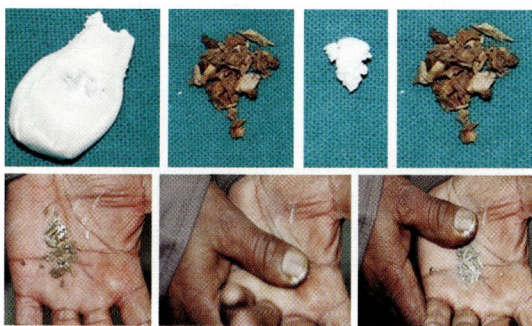

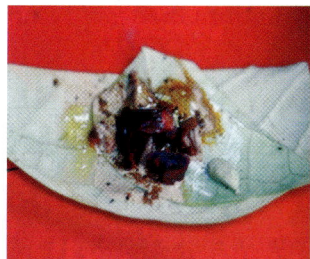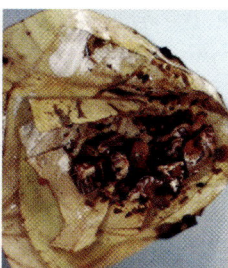

Fig. 2.16: A betel quid preparation consisting of areca nut, slaked lime, catechu, tobacco, elaichi, wrapped in a betel leaf.

Fig. 2.14: Conventional way of mixing/rubbing tobacco with slaked lime.

Another interesting, but a deadly form of tobacco use by population of Northern India was a dentifrice containing tobacco, marketed as *Musa ka gul*. A powdered form of tobacco that is applied on the teeth and gums and massaged *to clean one's teeth*.

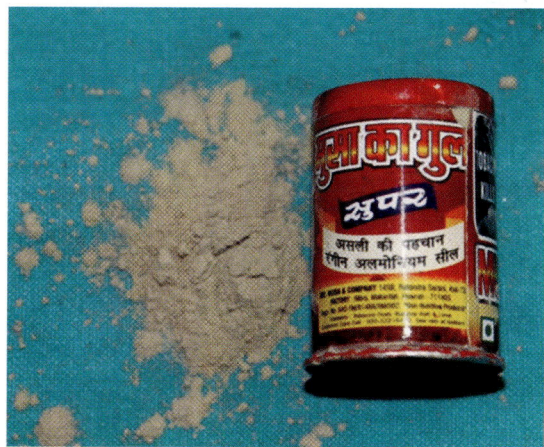

Fig. 2.15: Dentifrice containing tobacco used by the rural population in this region.

Betel Quid Preparation

The conventional method of consuming areca nut, slaked lime, catechu, tobacco, *elaichi*, wrapped in a betel leaf, known as pan, was also prevalent among the population of Northern India.

ADDITIONAL TOBACCO FORMS

SMOKE FORMS

Flavored and Herbal Bidis

Bidis sold in India are not flavored or typically packaged in packets, cones, cartons or tins as colorful as those found in the United States or Europe. Bidis exported for sale in the United States are available in brightly colored packages and a variety of flavors such as cherry, honey, strawberry, chocolate, mango, and lemon-lime. Packets and cones typically hold 20 Indian-style bidi cigarettes. They claim to contain mixtures of herbs rolled in tendu leaves and are marketed as safer, healthier alternatives to cigarettes. The flavoring of bidis has contributed to their popularity among youth and young adults.

In India, Dalmia Consumer Care recently launched a tobacco-less bidi 'Vardaan' which is meant to deliver safer alternative to the current bidi smoker. It claims to be "the world's first non-tobacco alternative that stimulates the pleasures of tobacco and mimics tobacco smoke". It has a mix of natural plants specially treated without chemicals and rolled in tendu leaf.

Chutta

Chuttas are coarsely prepared cheroots. They are usually the products of cottage and small-scale industries, or are made at home. Nearly 9% of the tobacco produced in India is used for making chuttas. This habit is widespread in the coastal areas of Andhra Pradesh, Tamil Nadu and Odisha.

Reverse Chutta Smoking

In Srikakulam, Andhra Pradesh the smoking of chuttas (coarsely prepared cigars) is the most prevalent habit. This habit's characteristic is putting the fired extreme of the cigarette inside the mouth, while the cigarette is being held by the teeth and lips, the seal provided the lips allows to slow inhaling of the cigarette.

Chillum

Chillum smoking is an exclusively male practice; it is limited to the Northern states of India, predominantly in rural areas. It involves smoking tobacco in a clay pipe that is 10–14 cm long. Chillum smoking requires deep pulmonary effect. This increases chance of oral cancer and lung cancer. They are made locally, are inexpensive and easily available. A chillum is shared by a group of individuals, so in addition to increasing their risk of cancer, people who share a chillum increase their chances of spreading colds, flu, and other lung illnesses. Chillum probably predates the introduction of tobacco to India and was used for smoking opium and other narcotics.

Dhumti

Unlike beedis and chuttas, dhumtis are not available from vendors but are prepared by

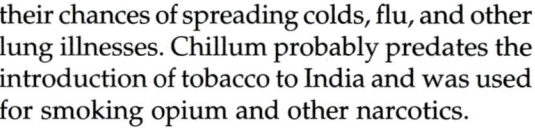

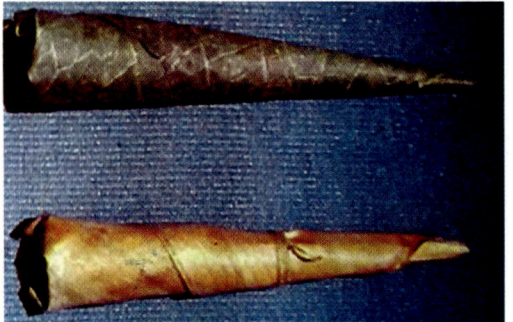

the smokers themselves. Dhumti is a kind of a conical cigar made by rolling tobacco leaf in the leaf of another plant. This form of smoking is more prevalent in Goa.

Pipe

Pipe smoking is one of the oldest forms of tobacco use. The different kinds of pipes used for smoking range from the small-stemmed European types made of wood to long-stemmed pipes made from metal or other material.

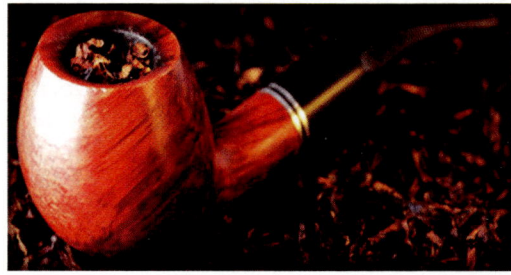

Hooklis

Hooklis are clay pipes commonly used in Western India. Once the pipe is lit, it is smoked intermittently. Hookli smoking was practised by men in the Bhavnagar district of Gujarat.

Smokeless Forms

The term smokeless tobacco is used to describe tobacco that is consumed without heating or burning at the time of use. Smokeless tobacco can be used orally or nasally. In the nasal use, a small quantity of very fine tobacco powder mixed with aromatic substances called dry snuff, is inhaled nasally. The oral use of smokeless tobacco is widely prevalent in India; the different methods of consumption include preparations are either placed in various parts of the mouth and sucked (dipping), chewing and applying tobacco preparations to the teeth and gums.

Gundi

Gundi is a mixture of cured tobacco, coriander seeds and other spices. Each constituent is fried separately, powdered coarsely and mixed and the product is scented with resinous oil. Gundi is known as *kadapan* in Odisha and Bengal; it is also used in Gujarat.

Zarda

Zarda is prepared by cutting tobacco leaves into small pieces and boiling them in water with slaked lime and spices until the water evaporates. It is then dried, and coloring and flavoring agents are added. It may be chewed by itself, with areca nut or in betel quid. It is available in small packets or tins.

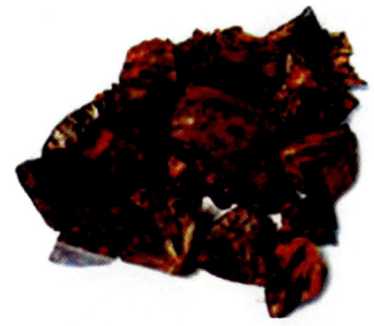

on the spot and chewed as a quid. Its use is becoming popular in Gujarat, especially among the youth.

Dry Snuff

It is a mixture of dried tobacco powder and some scented chemicals which is inhaled and is common in the elderly population of India. Snuff is responsible for cancers of the nose and jaw.

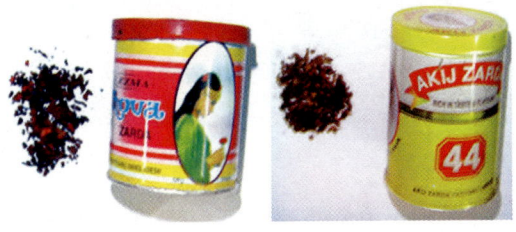

In India, it is used in two forms—pilapatti and kalipatti. Pilapatti is supposed to be milder in form, whereas kalipatti is supposed to be harder. Pilapatti look yellow in color and granules are fine, whereas kalipatti look black and granules are loose.

It is often used by men and women, of middle and upper socioeconomic groups as an ingredient in betel quid in India.

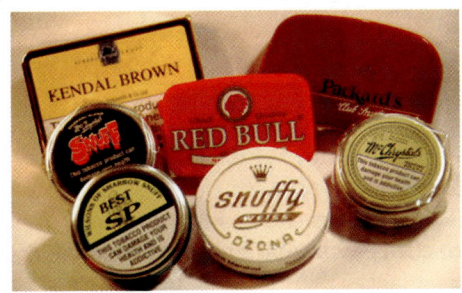

Kiwam

Kiwam is a thick tobacco paste; it is also available as granules or pellets. To prepare

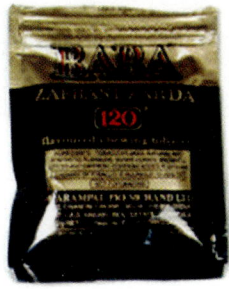

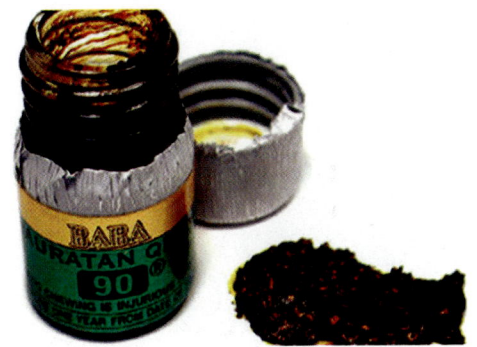

Mawa

Mawa is a preparation containing thin shavings of areca nut with the addition of some tobacco and slaked lime that is mixed

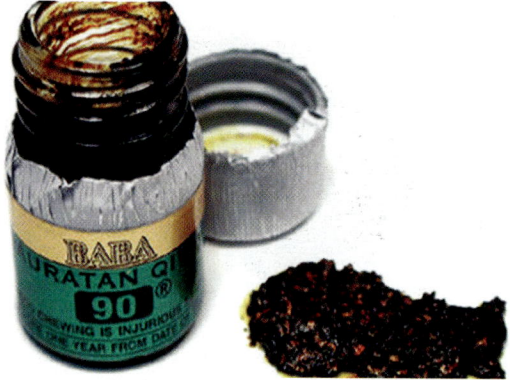

Mainpuri Tobacco

In the Mainpuri district of Uttar Pradesh and nearby areas, this preparation is very popular. It contains mainly tobacco with slaked lime, finely cut areca nut, camphor and cloves.

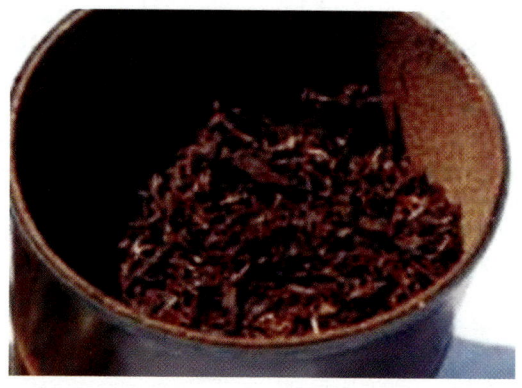

kiwam, the midribs and veins of tobacco leaves are removed, and the remaining matter is boiled in water. Powdered spices (saffron, cardamom, aniseed and musk) are added, and the mixture is stirred and allowed to macerate until it becomes a paste, from which granules and pellets are made. It is used by upper socioeconomic group of the population in India.

Snus

Swedish snuff called snus is available in tea bag like pouches. The pouch can be kept in the buccal or labial groove and sucked.

Hnatsay

Hnatsay is made by mixing the tobacco with honey or alcohol which is available in the market. It is used with betel quid. Different types of scents are added to it to give different flavors. It is available in either plastic bags or plastic glasses.

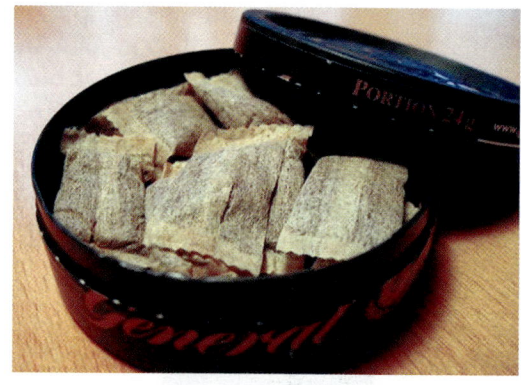

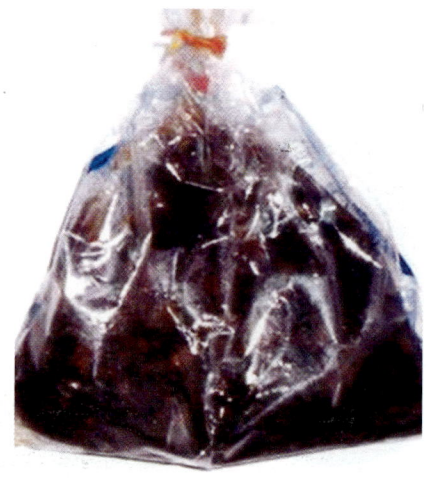

Dohra

Dohra is a wet mixture of tobacco, areca nut and other ingredients like catechu (kattha), pipermint, elaichi. It is mainly produced in Jaunpur district of Uttar Pradesh. It is marketed without any brand name and the name of manufacturer. Dohra is marketed in two ways; in one packet or in two packets. One packet is tobacco mixed and in two packets,

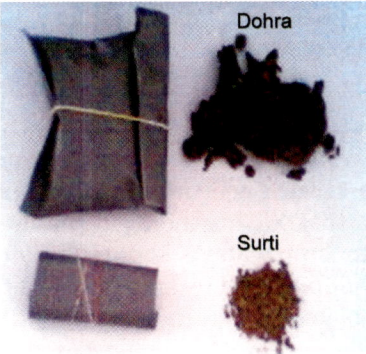

Dohra

Surti

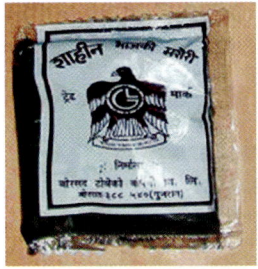 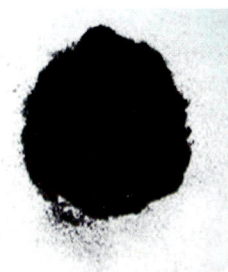

one contains mixtures other than tobacco and second one contains tobacco (zarda).

Applying Tobacco

Gudakhu

Gudakhu is a paste of tobacco and sugar molasses. It is available commercially and is carried in a metal container but can be made by the users themselves. It is commonly used in Bihar, Odisha, Uttar Pradesh and Uttaranchal. These preparations are commonly used by women and involve direct application of tobacco to the gums, thus increasing the risk of cancer of the gums.

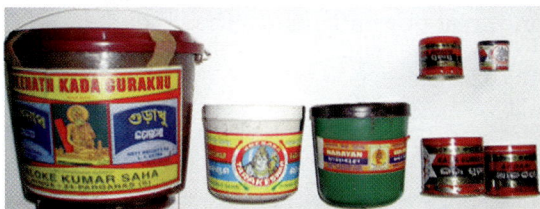

Mishri

Mishri is a roasted, powdered preparation made by baking tobacco on a hot metal plate until it is uniformly black, later on, it is powdered. Women, who use it to clean their teeth initially, soon apply mishri several times a day. Generally, it is carried in a small metal container; it is taken out with the index finger and applied to teeth and gums. This habit is common in Maharashtra and in Goa. It is applied to the teeth and gums, often for the

purpose of cleaning the teeth. Users then tend to hold it in their mouths (due to the nicotine addiction). Predominantly used by women, in lower socioeconomic groups.

Red Tooth Powder

It is commonly known as **Lal dantmanjan.** It is red colored tooth powder. In India, the misconception is widespread that tobacco is good for the teeth. This is commonly used in India. Many brands are available in Indian market. It is widely used by women and men, young, adults and kids.

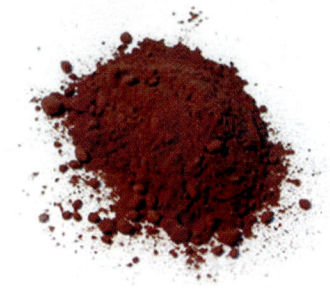

Creamy Snuff

Commercial preparations of tobacco paste are marketed in toothpaste-like tubes. They are advertised as possessing anti-bacterial activity and being good for the gums and teeth. These products are thus used like regular toothpaste, but users soon become addicted. This practice seems popular with children in Goa. Constituents of this paste are tobacco, clove oil, glycerine, spearmint, menthol and camphor. The manufacturer recommends letting the paste linger in the mouth before rinsing. It is primarily used by women. Creamy snuff is available in brand names: IPCO (Asha Industries product), Denobac, Tona, Ganesh, etc.

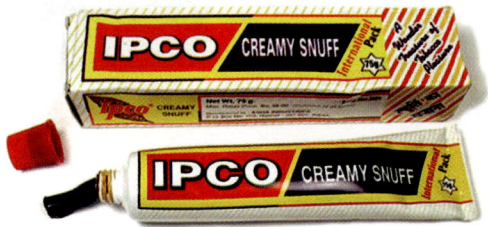

Bajjar

Bajjar is dry snuff (also known as tapkeer) applied commonly by women in Gujarat on the teeth and gums.

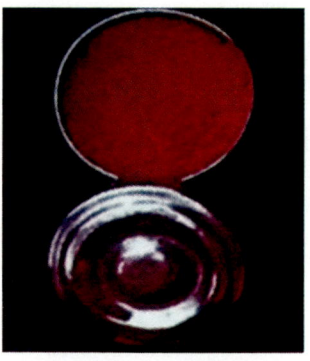

Sipping Tobacco

Tobacco Water

Tobacco water (known as *tuibur* in Mizoram and *hidakphu* in Manipur) is manufactured by passing tobacco smoke through water. It is sipped and retained in mouth for 5–10 minutes and then spat out. In general, in one sip usually 5–0 ml tobacco water is kept within mouth. It is either sipped directly from bottle or through cotton soaked with tobacco water.

The most important practical implication of knowing the various tobacco brands and practices in a population or region, for a clinician is, to elicit the history of the particular habit a patient has. This knowledge can be applied by professionals to know and understand tobacco habits in patients. For instance, to overcome a communication gap (language/physical and mental disabilities) between a doctor and his/her patient, the photographs or samples of tobacco brands can be shown. This will particularly help in knowing the culprit form of tobacco, establishing a rapport or striking a positive relationship with the patient. This practice would not only make us better clinicians/researchers, but also will help us understand and treat our patients well.

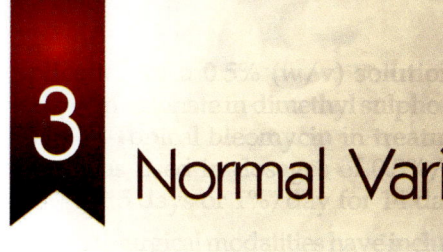

Normal Variations of the Oral Mucosa

Initial responsibility of differentiating harmless oral findings from those of tobacco induced almost always rests with a dentist. Distinguishing these signs at the earliest possible stage is essential. Thus, the normal variations of oral mucosa are shown, that may be seen more prominently in tobacco users and thus familiarity to these variations is important for a clinician.

BUCCAL MUCOSA

Linea Alba

It is derived from the Greek word which means "white line". It is a horizontal streak on the buccal mucosa at the level of the occlusal plane extending from retrocommissure to the posterior buccal mucosa.

Etiology

- Most likely associated with pressure, frictional irritation, or sucking trauma from the facial surfaces of the teeth.
- More prominent in individuals with reduced overjet of the posterior teeth.

Clinical Presentation

- It is usually present bilaterally.
- It is restricted to dentulous areas at the level of occlusal plane.
- It is often scalloped in shape.

Treatment

- No treatment is required.
- The horizontal white streak may disappear spontaneously in some people.

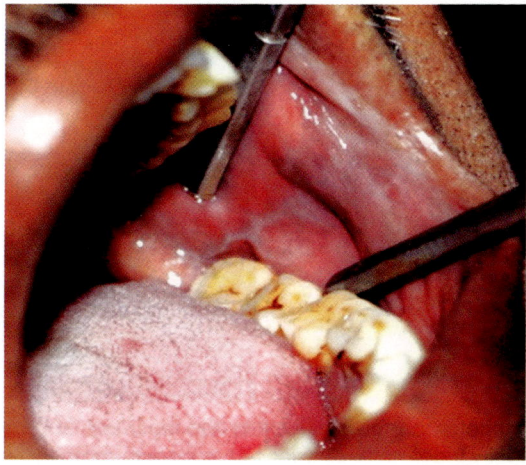
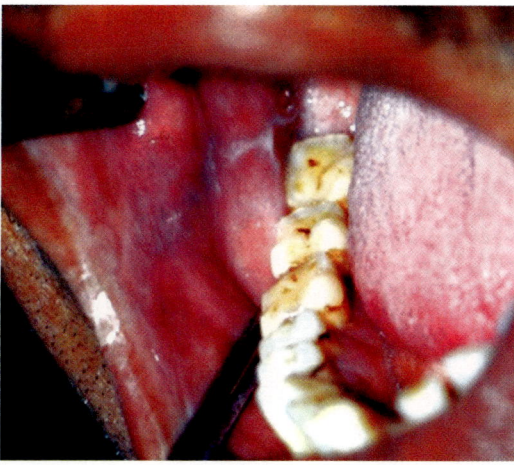

Fig. 3.1: Linea alba at the level of occlusal plane in young individuals with tobacco habits.

Fordyce Granules

They are ectopic sebaceous glands without hair follicles within the oral mucosa.

Etiology

They represent a developmental anomaly.

Completely asymptomatic and discovered on routine examination.

Clinical Presentation

- They present as multiple yellowish white papules.
- Often seen in aggregates or in confluent collections, most commonly on the buccal mucosa, vermilion border of the upper lip and retromolar region.
- Prevalence in adults ranges from 70 to 85%, with a slight predominance in men.

Treatment

- Usually no treatment is required.
- Tri chloroacetic acid (TCA) chemical peel
- Carbon dioxide laser
- Photodynamic therapy with 5-aminolevulinic acid
- Oral isotretinoin
- Curettage with electrocoagulation.

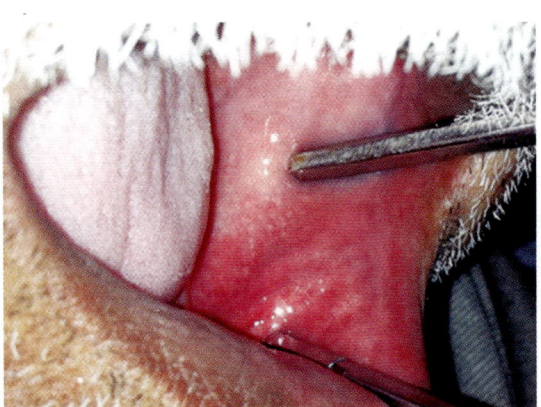

Fig. 3.2: Presence of ectopic collection of sebaceous glands on the left buccal mucosa in a 60-year-old male.

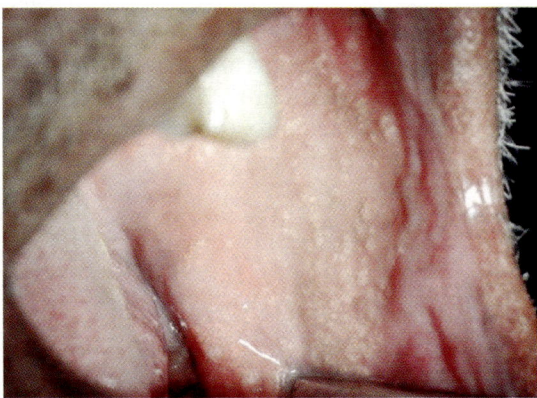

Fig. 3.3: Fordyce granules on the right buccal mucosa in a 70-year-old male patient.

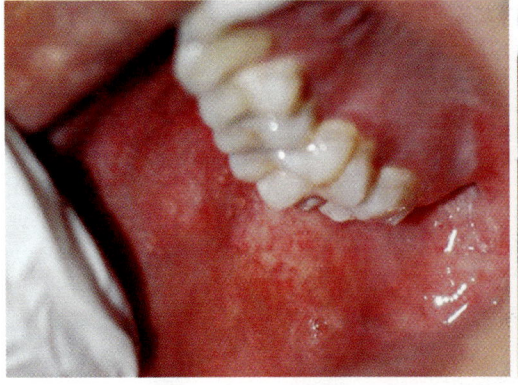
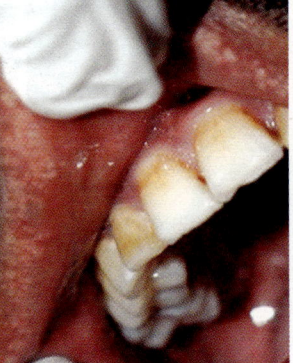
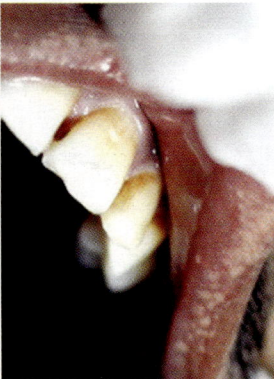

Fig. 3.4: Presence of Fordyce's granules on the right buccal mucosa, adjacent to the maxillary first molar tooth and on labial mucosa bilaterally near the vermilion border, in a 24-year-old male with cigarette and gutkha chewing habits.

Leukoedema

It is a common mucosal alteration that represents a variation of the normal condition rather than a true pathologic condition.

Features

- Most frequent site is the buccal mucosa, present bilaterally.

- It usually has a faint, white, diffuse, and filmy appearance, with numerous surface folds resulting in the wrinkling of the mucosa.
- It cannot be scrapped off, and it disappears or fades upon stretching the mucosa.

Treatment

- No treatment is indicated.
- There are no malignant changes reported with this lesion.

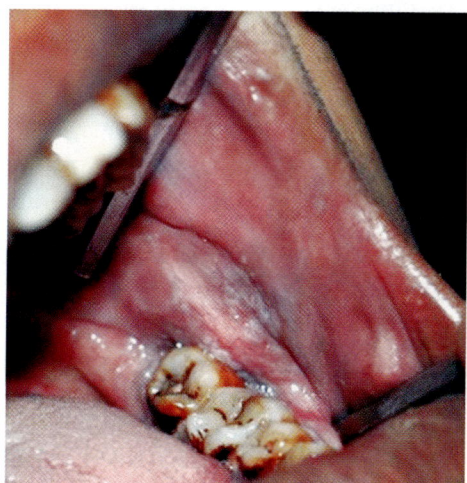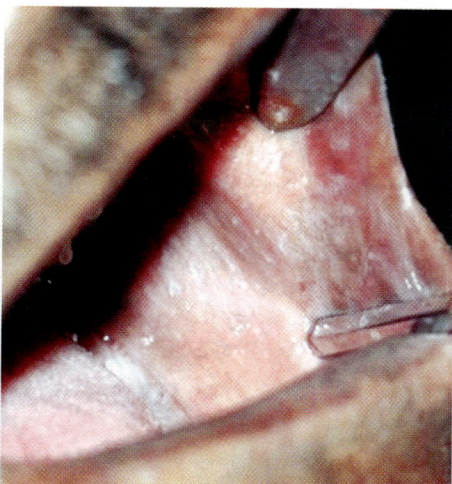

Fig. 3.5: A 50-year-old male with bidi and cigarette smoking habits presented with leukoedema on the left buccal mucosa.

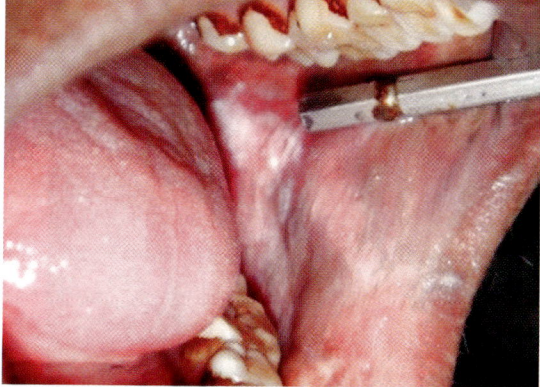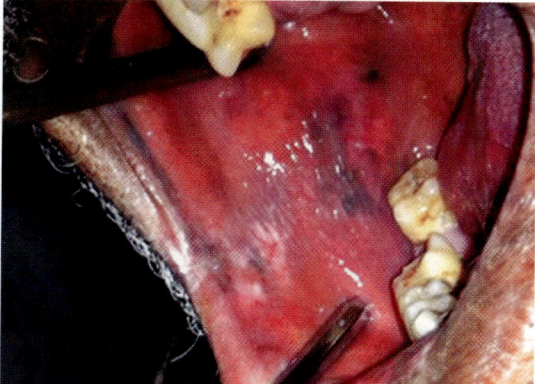

Fig. 3.6: A non-scrapable white patch that disappears on stretching the left buccal mucosa of a 50-year-old male patient, with bidi smoking habit.

Fig. 3.7: Leukoedema on the right buccal mucosa in a 54-year-old male with bidi smoking habits.

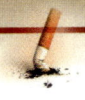

Purpura

Purpura refers to purple-colored spots and patches that occur on the skin, organs, and in mucous membranes, including the lining of the mouth. Purpura occurs when small blood vessels join together or leak blood under the skin.

Etiology

The purpuric macule is produced by a blunt traumatic insult to the skin or mucosa of sufficient force to cause the discharge of blood on the surface.

Clinical Presentation

- Purpuric areas are quite red. If sufficient time has lapsed to permit some breakdown of the hemoglobin pigment, the "bruise" is bluish, undergoing the color changes from green to yellow.
- The size of the purpuric macule varies according to the size and the force of the physical agent inflicting the damage.
- The most common sites are the palate, the cheek, and the floor of the mouth.
- Diascopy (is using a glass slide to apply pressure to the area of concern) test is

negative. The lesion does not blanch on pressure because the red blood cells are within the tissues rather than in vessels.

Treatment

Removing devices that are causing the trauma and rechecking the patient to make sure the lesions have resolved is necessary.

TONGUE

Hypertrophy of Circumvallate Papillae

Papillitis refers to inflammation of the papillae, and sometimes the term hypertrophy is used interchangeably.

Etiology

This may occur due to mechanical irritation, or as a reaction to an upper respiratory tract infection.

Clinical Presentation

Hypertrophic circumvallate papillae may be seen as pale pink papules on the posterior surface of dorsum of tongue. They are usually asymptomatic and require no intervention. A normal anatomic variation of the papillae of tongue, more commonly seen in tobacco users.

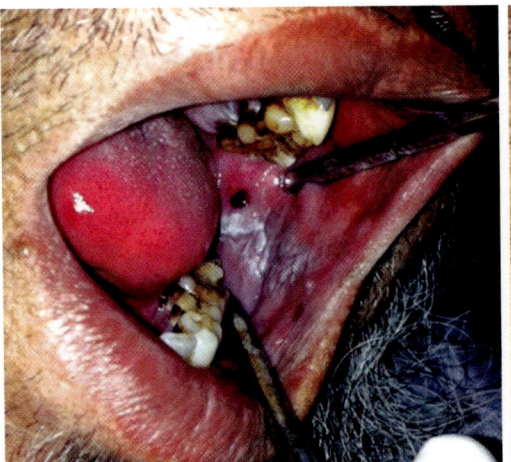
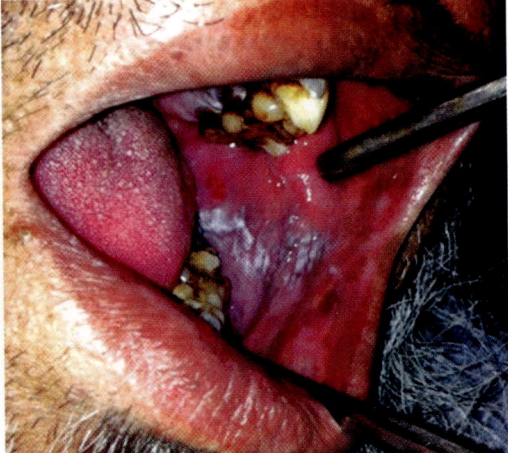

Fig. 3.8: Presence of purpuric spot, due to trauma, along with homogenous leukoplakia on the left buccal mucosa in a 58-year-old male patient with bidi and hookah smoking habits.

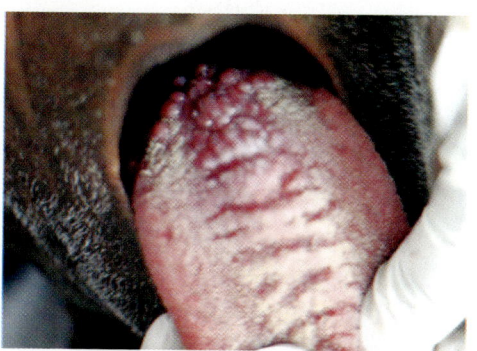

Fig. 3.9: Hypertrophic papillae and fissures on the posterior-dorsal aspect of tongue, in a 58-year-old bidi smoker.

Geographic Tongue

Geographic tongue, also known as erythema migrans and benign migratory glossitis, is a condition of unknown cause. It is seen in association with fissured tongue, but is inversely associated with smoking.

Etiology

- Association between certain types of psoriasis and geographic tongue is present.
- Psychological conditions
- It has been seen with increased frequency in patients with pernicious anemia.
- In pregnant patients, where it is possibly associated with folic acid deficiency or hormonal fluctuations.

- Gastrointestinal disturbances
- Candidiasis

Clinical Presentation

It is characterized by presence of atrophic patches surrounded by elevated keratotic margins. The desquamated areas appear red and may be slightly tender. The patterns change, when followed over a period of weeks or months, giving rise to serpeginous white lines, running across the dorsum of tongue.

Treatment

- Most patients require no definitive treatment.
- Observation and reassurance of the patient.
- For symptomatic geographic tongue, supportive and symptomatic management include bland diet, plenty of fluids.
- Multivitamin
- Acetaminophen for systemic pain relief
- Topical anesthetic agent such as viscous lidocaine or benzydamine (tantum)—rinse for local pain relief.
- Antihistamine, such as diphenhydramine (Benadryl) should be used.
- If the lesions do not respond to antihistamine/supportive/symptomatic therapy, then a corticosteroid, such as betamethasone can be used as a rinse for a few minutes and swallowed, twice daily for 7 to 14 days.

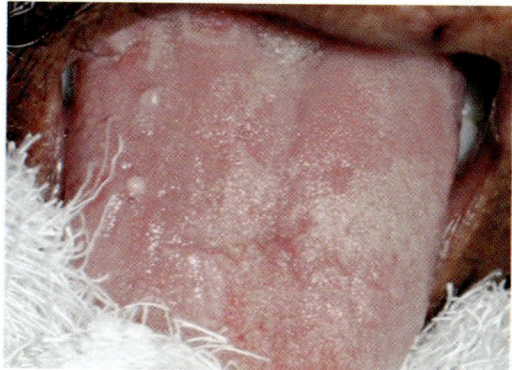

Fig. 3.10: Atrophic patches surrounded by elevated keratotic margins, on the dorsum of tongue in a 60-year-old male patient.

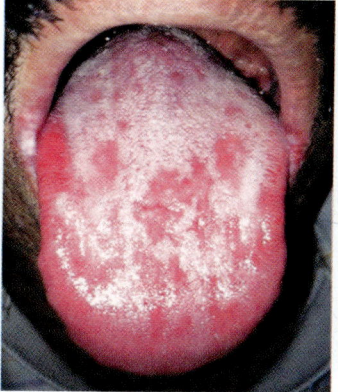

Fig. 3.11: De-papillated areas on the dorsum of tongue in a 60-year-old male patient.

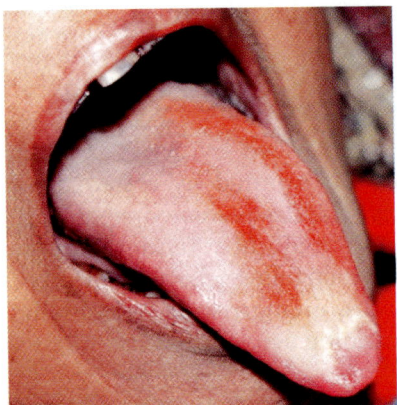

Fig. 3.12: Pan stains and geographic tongue in a 50-year-old male patient with pan chewing habit.

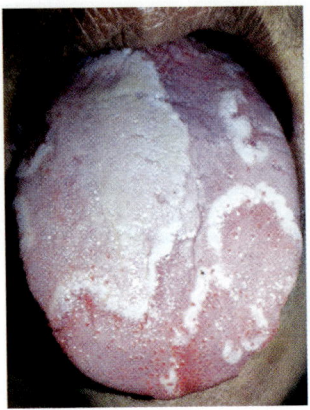

Fig. 3.13: Irregular thick white serpiginous lines on the dorsum of tongue in a 58-year-old male smoker.

Fissured Tongue

It is characterized by presence of numerous grooves, or fissures, on the dorsal tongue surface. It may be seen in association with geographic tongue and more common in people who have glossitis or geographic tongue.

Etiology

It is developmental in origin.

Clinical Presentation

It is characterized by deep, branching grooves along its top surface, instead of just the midline groove. It can occur at any age, although the fissures tend to increase and deepen with age.

This deepening causes the trapping of food debris and desquamated epithelial cells within the grooves.

Usually, it is asymptomatic but bacterial or fungal infection can cause soreness or burning sensation on tongue. When this occurs, the grooves become red and prominent. There is shedding of adjacent papillae resulting in an inflamed appearance of tongue.

Treatment

• Usually no treatment is required.
• Gently brushing the dorsal surface of tongue is recommended to prevent accumulation of food debris.

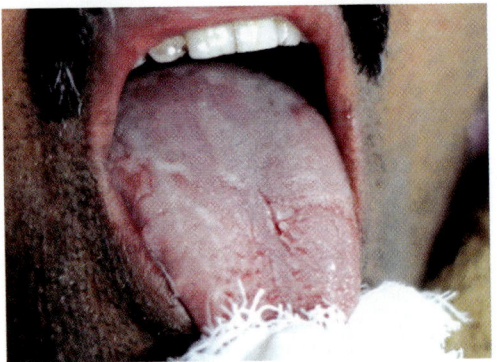

Fig. 3.14: A 45-year-old male with tobacco chewing habit presented with cracks/fissures on the dorsal aspect of tongue.

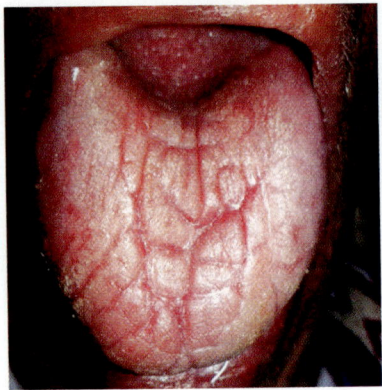

Fig. 3.15: Numerous fissures on the dorsal surface of tongue in a 58-year-old bidi smoker.

4 Adverse Effects of Tobacco

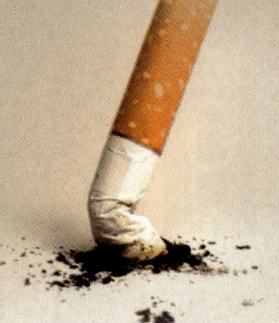

Tobacco a transitory pleasure; that invites a future of disease, death and horror

EFFECTS ON GENERAL HEALTH

1. *Brain*: Strokes
2. *Skin, eye and ear diseases*: Psoriasis, cataract, macular degeneration, ear infections
3. *Respiratory infection*: Cancer, tuberculosis, asthma, COPD, interstitial lung disease
4. *Bones*: Brittle bones, osteoporosis
5. *Immune system*: Reduced immune response, increased infection
6. *Pregnancy and babies*: Miscarriages, stillbirths, preterm delivery, low birth weight, sudden infant death syndrome, and developmental impairments
7. *Physical appearance*: Premature aging, alopecia, tooth decay
8. *Oro-pharynx/larynx*: Inflammation, ulcers, precancerous and cancers
9. *Heart and circulatory system*: Hypertension, heart disease, heart attacks, coronary and other artery disease, and peripheral vascular disease
10. *Cancers*: Pancreas, kidney, and urinary bladder
11. Sexual and reproductive system: Erectile dysfunction (men), impaired menstrual cycle, early menopause (women), reduced fertility, and cancers.

EFFECTS ON ORAL HEALTH

1. Leukoedema
2. Pan encrustation and stains
3. Tobacco-lime user's lesion
4. Tobacco pouch keratosis
5. Chewer's mucosa
6. Central papillary atrophy of the tongue
7. Palatal erythema
8. Nicotinic stomatitis
9. Pre-leukoplakia
10. Lichenoid reaction
11. Homogenous leukoplakia
12. Speckled leukoplakia
13. Candidal leukoplakia
14. Verrucous leukoplakia
15. Oral submucous fibrosis
16. Carcinoma

EFFECTS ON DENTAL HEALTH

1. Extrinsic stains on teeth
2. Wasting diseases of teeth
3. Gingivitis and periodontitis

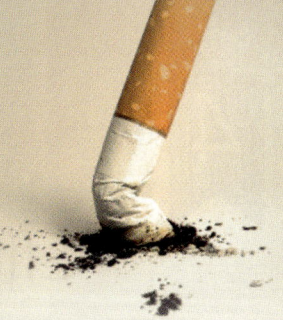

5 Tobacco Associated Oral Mucosal Lesions

Tobacco surely was designed "To poison and destroy mankind"

A variety of tobacco associated lesions has been reviewed and categorized because of their possible causal association with oral cancer and various potentially malignant disorders.

An international working group comprising specialists in the fields of epidemiology, oral medicine and pathology and molecular biology with a special interest in oral cancer and precancer met in London in May 2005 to discuss current concepts, the terminology, classifications, the natural history, pathology and of molecular markers and to critically analyse the evolution of knowledge and practice concerning the diagnosis and management of what have been called, collectively, precancerous lesions and conditions of the oral mucosa. The workshop was coordinated by the WHO Collaborating Centre for Oral Cancer and Precancer in the UK.

The terms 'pre-cancer', 'precursor lesions', pre-malignant', 'intra epithelial neoplasia' and 'potentially malignant' have been used in the international literature to broadly describe clinical presentations that may have a potential to become cancer. They all convey the concept of a two-step or multi-step process of cancer development, but it is unlikely, on priori grounds, that there is uniformity in the way individual patients or tissues behave. The latest WHO monograph on head and neck tumours (2005) uses the term 'epithelial precursor lesions'.

The consensus of the present working group was to recommend the term 'potentially malignant disorders', as it conveys that not all lesions and conditions described under this term may transform to cancer, amongst which some may have an increased potential for malignant transformation.

The lesions and conditions recorded will reflect the range of conditions and diseases found in our survey population in "Northern India, Uttar Pradesh" with "India".

BUCCAL MUCOSA

Chemical Burn

The habit of placement of khaini (tobacco in combination with lime) produces a yellow-white plaque at the site of placement of this product. As the consumption of this form of tobacco is not uncommon, this lesion is often seen in the population of Northern India. The mixture is usually placed in contact with the labial/buccal mucosa and/or vestibular region.

Clinical Presentation

The lesion may mimic a leukoplakia, which is a non-scrapable patch/plaque and thus must be distinguished from a chemical burn, which can easily be scraped off with the help of a gauze piece.

Treatment

Usually, cessation of the habit will restore the normal mucosal characteristics. In case the

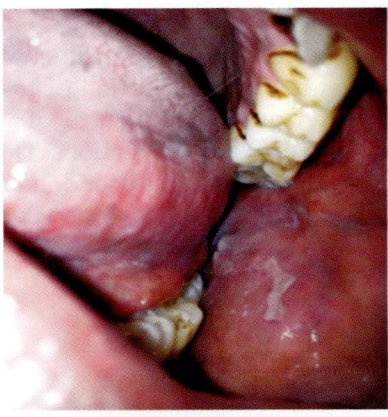 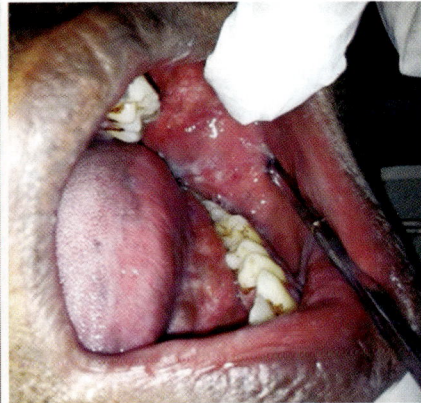

Fig. 5.1: A scrapable white patch seen on the left buccal mucosa of a 37-year-old male patient with a habit of chewing tobacco mixed with slaked lime.

lesion does not resolve despite cessation of habit, a biopsy must be performed and treatment planning must be altered depending on the results of the biopsy.

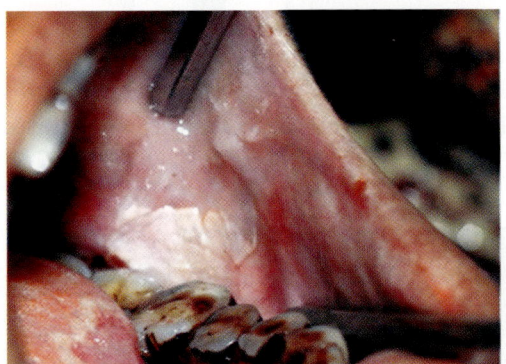

Fig. 5.2: Presence of a scrapable white patch on the left buccal mucosa of 48-year-old male patient with habit of chewing tobacco with slaked lime.

Tobacco Pouch Keratosis

Another specific tobacco-related oral mucosal alteration that occurs in association with smokeless tobacco use either from snuff or chewing tobacco.

Clinical Presentation

Such lesions typically occur in the buccal or labial vestibule where the tobacco is held, but they can also extend onto the adjacent gingiva

and buccal mucosa. Early lesions may show slight wrinkling that disappears when the tissues are stretched. It must be differentiated from a leukoplakic patch that is usually thick and shows a characteristic cracked-mud appearance.

Treatment

Discontinuation of tobacco use usually reverts the alteration of mucosa caused by it.

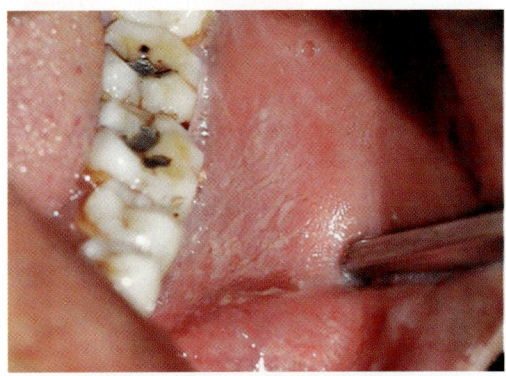

Fig. 5.3: A wrinkled white patch on the left buccal vestibular region, in a 24-year-old male with tobacco chewing habit.

Smoker's Melanosis

Smoker's melanosis refers to the pigmented oral mucosal sites associated with smoke-forms of tobacco, such as bidi, cigarette, and hookah among many others. It is reputed to be the most common smoked-tobacco related oral mucosal lesion, with a reported prevalence of 11.8%.

Clinical Presentation

It is characterized by discrete or coalescing multiple brown macules that usually involve the attached mandibular gingiva on the labial side, although pigmentation of the palate and buccal mucosa has also been associated with pipe smoking.

Treatment

A gradual return to normal pigmentation over several months to years has been reported following smoking cessation.

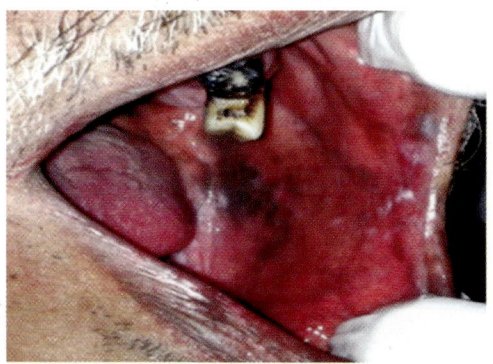

Fig. 5.4: A 60-year-old male patient with diffused melanin pigmentation on the left buccal mucosa with habit of bidi smoking.

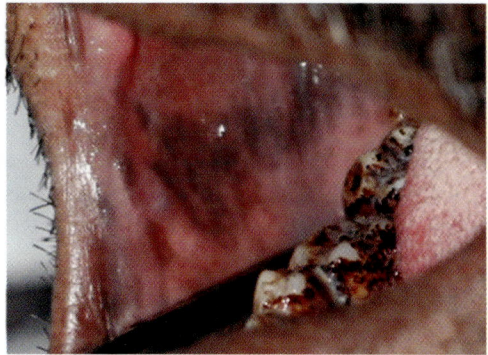

Fig. 5.5: Melanin pigmentation on the right buccal mucosa in a 50-year-old male associated with bidi smoking.

Pan Encrustation and Stains

A condition of the oral mucosa that shows evidence of incorporation of the ingredients of betel quid in the form of yellowish or reddish brown encrustations. The underlying areas may assume a pseudomembranous or wrinkled appearance. This type of lesion is seen frequently in pan chewers. The most common sites are buccal mucosa, labial mucosa and tongue.

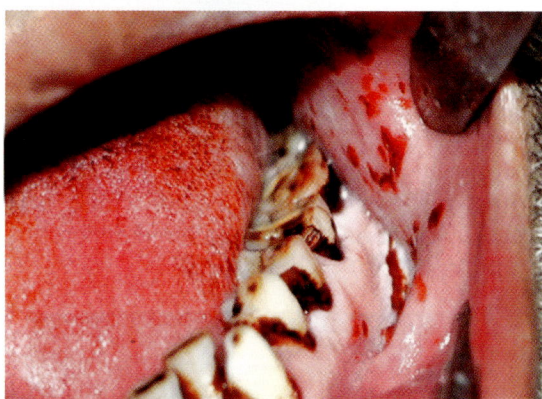

Fig. 5.6: Pan encrustation seen on the left buccal mucosa of a 55-year-old male patient with pan chewing habit.

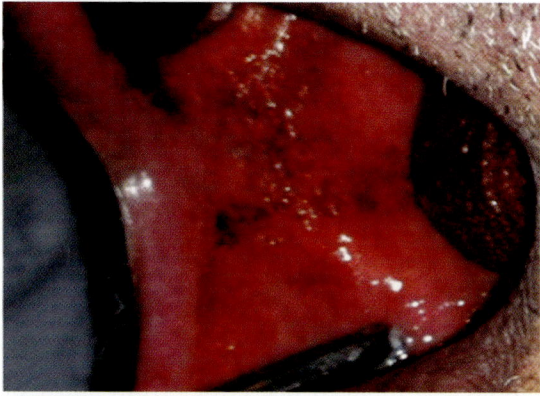

Fig. 5.7: Pan stains seen on buccal mucosa in a 54-year-old pan chewer.

Chewer's Mucosa

In chronic chewers a condition known as betel chewer's mucosa, a discoloured areca nut-encrusted change, is often found where the quid particles are retained. A condition of the oral mucosa in which, because of either direct action of the quid or the traumatic effect of chewing (or both), there is a tendency for the oral mucosa to desquamate or peel. The prevalence varies between 0.2% and 60% in different studies from South and Southeast Asia. Women are more frequently affected than men.

Clinical Presentation

Loose and detached white tags of tissue can also be seen and felt. The underlying areas may assume a pseudomembranous or wrinkled appearance. The area may also show evidence of incorporation of the quid ingredients in the form of yellowish or reddish brown encrustations. This type of lesion should be distinguished from cheek-biting, which is unintentional typically occurs in younger people, around 20–35 years.

Treatment

Cessation of habit will revert the normal appearance of oral mucosa gradually.

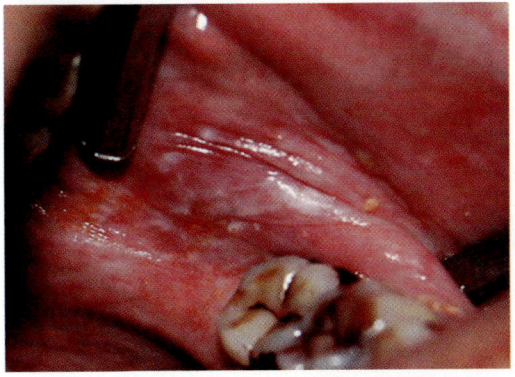

Fig. 5.8: Chewer's mucosa on the left buccal mucosa in a 35-year-old male with zarda and pan chewing habits.

Irritation Hyperplasia

Reactive lesions are tumor-like hyperplasia produced in association with chronic local irritation or trauma. Tobacco acts as a locally irritative agent causing hyperkeratinization and hyperplasia of the oral epithelium.

Clinical Presentation

It appears as a proliferative growth/outgrowth of the oral mucosal tissues, most commonly seen on the buccal mucosa and palate. It must be distinguished from any other source of irritation or mechanical trauma such as a sharp tooth, dentures, cheek biting; at the site of the lesion.

Treatment

Surgical excision of the growth is required along with refrainment from the cause of irritation.

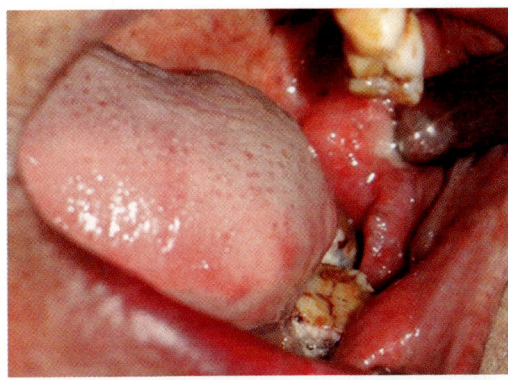

Fig. 5.9: Irritation hyperplasia on the left posterior buccal mucosal region a 40-year-old female patient with a habit of chewing pan.

Lichenoid Reaction

A lesion resembling oral lichen planus, seen exclusively among smokeless tobacco users. It usually occurs at the site of placement of tobacco. It has a reported prevalence of 2.2%.

Clinical Presentation

It is characterized by the presence of fine, white, wavy, parallel lines that do not overlap or criss-cross, are non-elevated, and in some instances radiate from a central erythematous area. A different natural history and a known history of tobacco use, along with the above clinical features may help differentiate lichenoid reaction from lichen planus.

Treatment

There may be complete regression when the causative habit is given up.

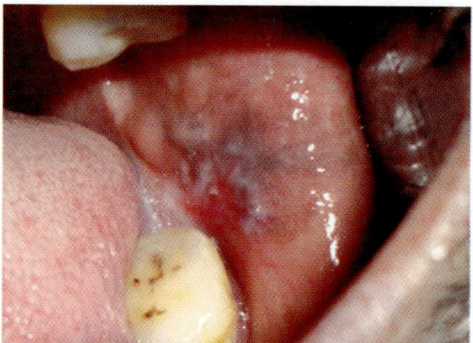

Fig. 5.10: Presence of an erythematous area with radiating white striae on the left buccal mucosa, posterior to the second molar tooth associated with gutkha chewing.

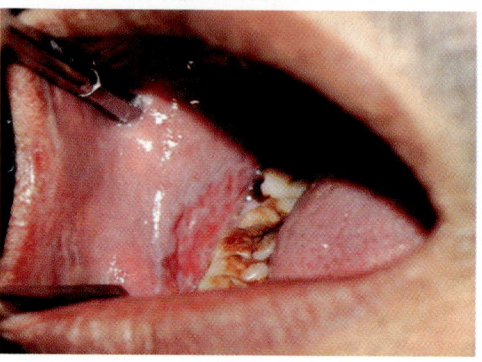

Fig. 5.11: Presence of erythematous area interspersed with white striae on the right lower posterior buccal mucosal region.

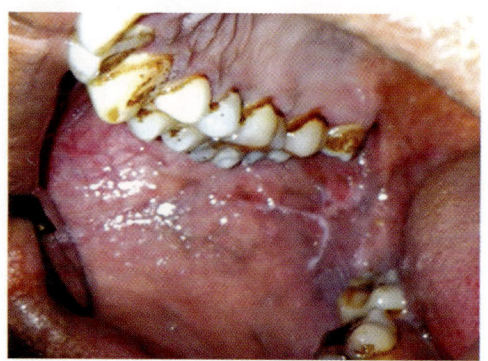

Fig. 5.12: A 40-year-old male presented with white striae on the right posterior region of buccal mucosa with the habit of gutkha chewing.

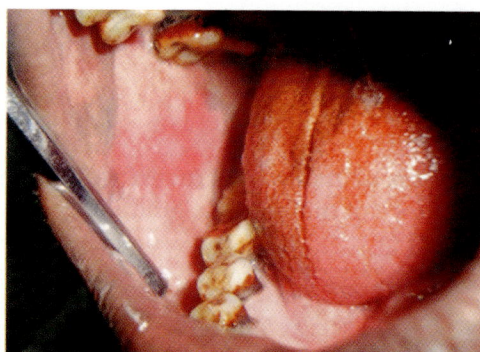

Fig. 5.13: Lichenoid reaction on the right buccal mucosa in a patient with pan chewing habit, associated with pan stains on the dorsum of tongue.

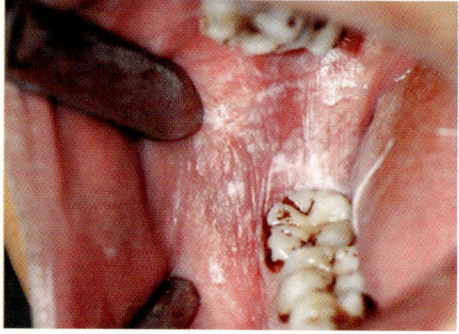

Fig. 5.14: A 25-year-old male with pan chewing habit presented with lichenoid reaction on the right posterior buccal mucosa.

Pre-leukoplakia

A pre-leukoplakia, conceived as a precursor stage of leukoplakia, defined as a low grade or very mild reaction of the mucosa. It is found that the mixed habit group of bidi smoking and tobacco chewing has the highest prevalence (6.1%) of pre-leukoplakia.

Clinical Presentation

It appears as a grey or greyish-white, but never completely white, area with a slight lobular pattern and with indistinct borders blending into the adjacent normal mucosa. They are most commonly seen on buccal mucosa.

Treatment

The pre-leukoplakias have showed a marked tendency to regress; in a very few patients pre-leukoplakia may turn into carcinoma.

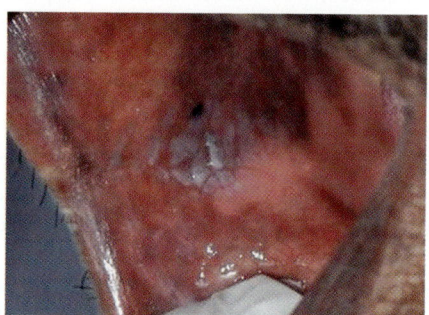

Fig. 5.15: Pre-leukoplakia on the right anterior buccal mucosa in a 63-year-old male patient with bidi smoking habit.

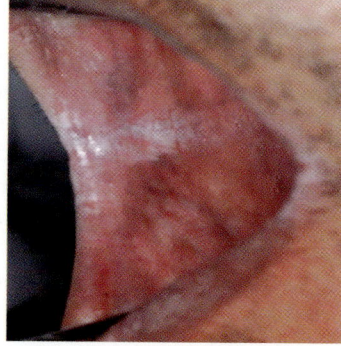

Fig. 5.16: Pre-leukoplakia on the left buccal mucosa in a 48-year-old male patient with bidi smoking habit.

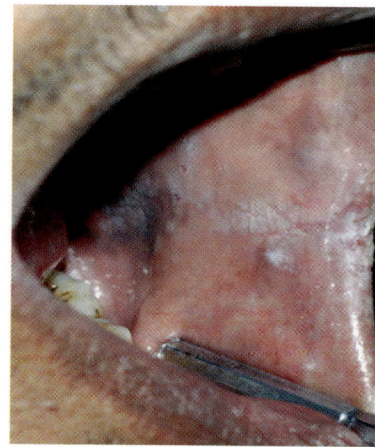

Fig. 5.17: A 50-year-old bidi smoker presented with a thin grey patch on the left buccal mucosa, with a characteristic cracked-mud appearance.

Leukoplakia

Leukoplakia (white patch) is defined as a predominantly white lesion of the oral mucosa that cannot be characterized as any other definable lesion. It is the most common precancerous lesion, and it occurs six times more commonly among smokers than non-smokers.

Two main clinical types of leukoplakia are recognized, being homogenous and non-homogenous leukoplakia. The distinction of these is purely clinical. Homogenous lesions are uniformly flat, thin and exhibit shallow cracks of the surface keratin. Non-homogenous varieties include:

- *Speckled*: Mixed, white and red, but retaining predominantly white character;
- *Nodular*: Small polypoid outgrowths, rounded red or white excrescences;
- *Verrucous*: Wrinkled or corrugated surface appearance.

Global prevalence is estimated to range from 0.5 to 3.4%. The point prevalence is estimated to be 2.6% (95% CI 1.72–2.74) with a reported rate of malignant transformation ranging from 0.13 to 17.5%. Various non-surgical and surgical treatments have been reported, but currently there is no consensus on the most appropriate one. Randomized controlled trials for non-surgical treatment show no evidence of effective prevention of malignant transformation and recurrence. Conventional surgery has its own limitations with respect to the size and site of the lesion but laser surgery has shown some encouraging results. There is no universal consensus on the duration or interval of follow-up of patients with the condition. The vast majority of potentially malignant disorders (PMD) in which oral squamous cell carcinoma develop are non-homogenous although 5% of homogenous PMD will develop carcinoma.

Clinical Presentation

The most common site affected is buccal mucosa (25%), mandibular gingiva (20%), tongue (10%), floor of the mouth (10%) and other oral sites account for the remainder.

Treatment

- Cessation of tobacco use and regular follow-up of the patient.
- **Carotenoids**
  1. **Beta-carotene:** It is a carotenoid commonly found in dark green, orange or yellowish vegetables, such as spinach, carrots, sweet potato, mango, papaya, and oranges. It is a vitamin A precursor. The use of beta-carotene has been recommended in order to prevent oral lesions (OL) and possibly oral cancer. The potential benefits and protective effects against cancer are possibly related to its antioxidizing action. This function is accomplished through a ligation between beta-carotene and oxygen, which is an unstable reactive molecule, thus diminishing the damaging effects of free radicals.
  Dose: 20 to 90 mg/day of beta-carotene in time periods from 3 to 12 months.
  2. **Lycopene:** It is a carotenoid without provitamin A action. This is a fat-soluble red pigment found in some fruits and vegetables. The greatest known source of lycopene is tomatoes. It has a uncommon feature of becoming bound to chemical species that react to oxygen, thus being the most efficient biological antioxidizing agent. The time period was three months, the dosages regimes from 4 to 8 mg/day.

- **Vitamins**
  1. **L-ascorbic acid (vitamin C):** L-ascorbic acid (L-AA), the so-called vitamin C, is found in citrous fruits such as kiwi, strawberries, papaya, and mango. Daily allowance for ascorbic and acid ranges between 100 and 120 mg/per day for adults. L-AA has antioxidizing properties and reacts with superoxide produced as a result of the cells' normal metabolic processes; this inactivation of superoxide inhibits the formation of nitrosamines during protein digestion and helps avoid damage to DNA and cellular protein.

  2. **α-Tocoferol (vitamin E):** α-Tocoferol (AT) is the commonest and most active form of vitamin E. It is found in plant oil, margarine and green leaves. The recommended daily limit rates are 10 mg/day for adult men and 8 mg/day for adult women. Tocoferol is an effective antioxidant at high levels of oxygen, protecting cellular membranes from lipidic peroxidation.

  3. **Retinoic acid (vitamin A):** Retinoic acid is obtained from carotene and animal products such as meat, milk, and eggs, which, while in the intestine, are converted, respectively, into retinal and retinol. 13-cRA is the retinoid recommended for OL treatment. The use of 13-cRA has been shown to be effective in resolving OL. Topical use of 0.1% isotretinoin gel also proved to be effective in resolution of oral leukoplakia.

  4. **Bleomycin:** Bleomycin is a cytotoxic antibiotic. OL were treated by the daily

application of a 0.5% (w/v) solution of bleomycin sulphate in dimethyl sulphoxide (DMSO). Topical bleomycin in treatment of OL was used in dosages of 0.5%/day for 12 to 15 days or 1%/day for 14 days.

Traditional surgical modalities have included mucosal resection by means of so-called "stripping" with graft coverage, usually an autologous skin graft. Alternatives to scalpel or standard excisional surgery include cryosurgery and use of laser ablation.

Homogenous Leukoplakia

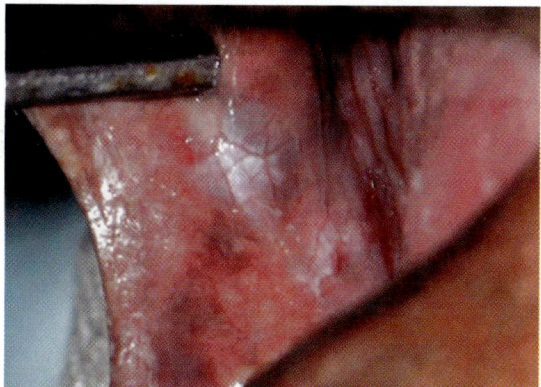

Fig. 5.18: Homogenous leukoplakia on the right buccal mucosa of a 55-year-old male patient with bidi smoking habit.

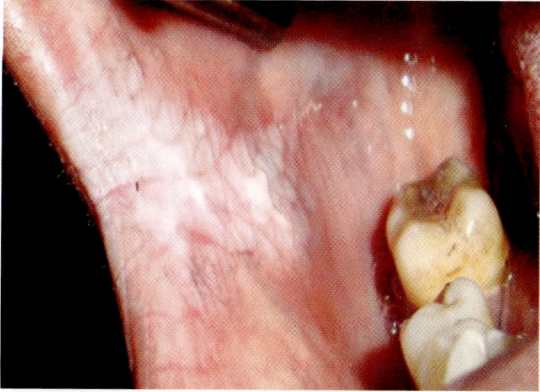

Fig. 5.19: Homogenous leukoplakia on the anterior right buccal mucosa of a 44-year-old male patient with bidi smoking habit.

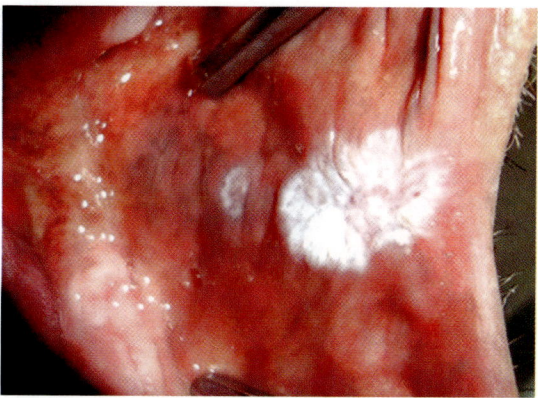

Fig. 5.20: Homogenous leukoplakia on the anterior region of left buccal mucosa in a 54-year-old male patient with bidi smoking habit.

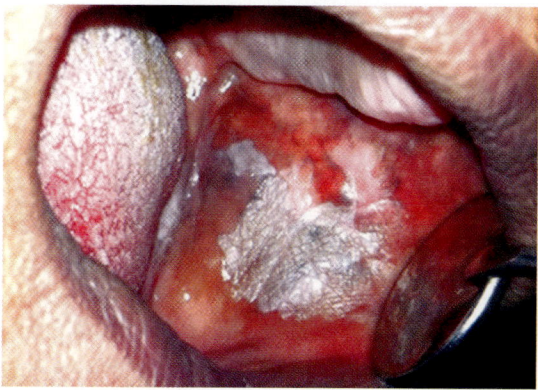

Fig. 5.21: Homogenous leukoplakia on the left buccal mucosa of a 36-year-old male patient with bidi smoking habit.

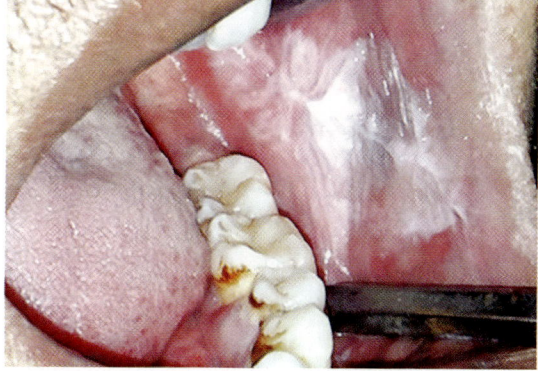

Fig. 5.22: Presence of a thickened white patch on left buccal mucosa in a 34-year-old male tobacco chewer.

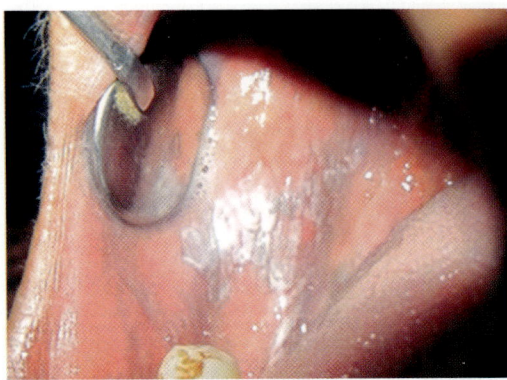

Fig. 5.23: Homogenous leukoplakia on the right buccal mucosa of a 56-year-old male patient with bidi smoking habit.

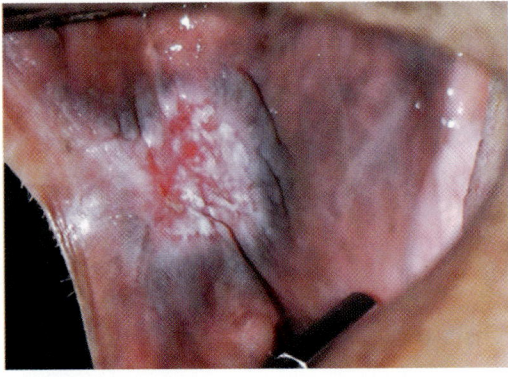

Fig. 5.26: Presence of a small erythematous patch surrounded by a white area along with diffused melanin pigmentation on the left buccal mucosa of a 46-year-old male patient with bidi smoking habit.

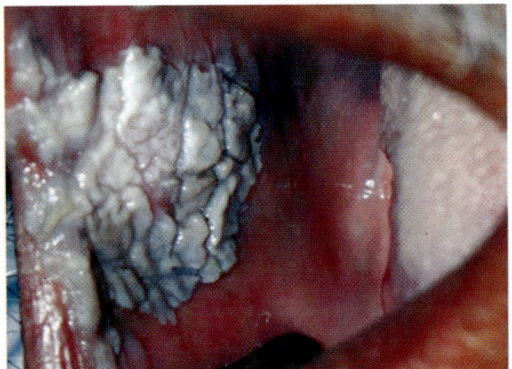

Fig. 5.24: Homogenous leukoplakia covering the right buccal mucosa in a 55-year-old male patient with bidi smoking habit.

Speckled Leukoplakia

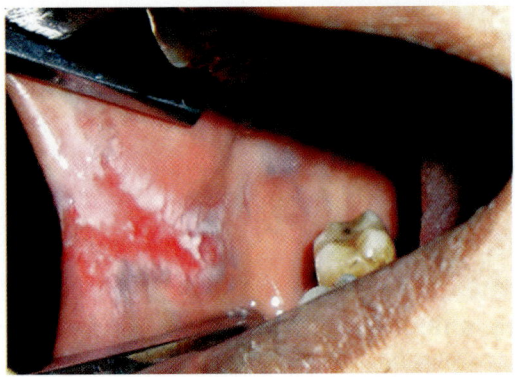

Fig. 5.27: Presence of a fiery red and white patch on the right anterior region of buccal mucosa in a 56-year-old bidi smoker.

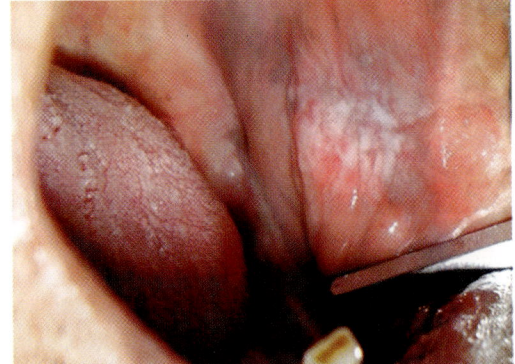

Fig. 5.25: Speckled leukoplakia on the left buccal mucosa of a 56-year-old male patient with bidi smoking habit.

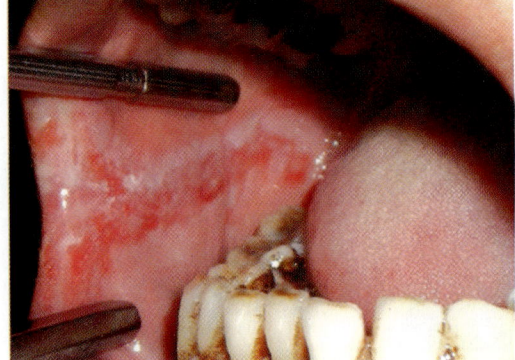

Fig. 5.28: A 48-year-old male patient with bidi smoking habit presented with an erythematous area covering the entire width of right buccal mucosa.

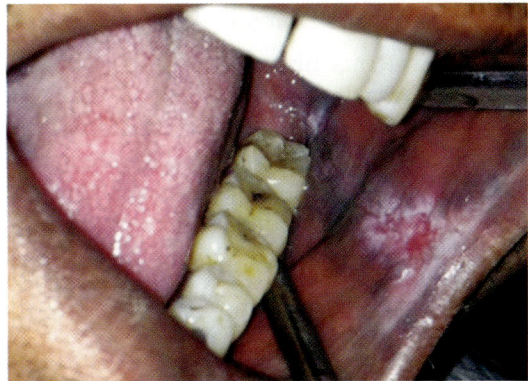

Fig. 5.29: Speckled leukoplakia involving the left anterior buccal mucosa in a 37-year-old male smoker.

Candidal Leukoplakia

Lehner (1964, 1967) recognized the presentation of chronic candidal infection in the form of leukoplakia and introduced the term "candidal leukoplakia". The terms "chronic hyperplastic candidosis" (CHC) and "candidal leukoplakia" (CL) appear to have been synonymously used until the mid-1980s.

Clinical Presentation

The most common and arguably the classic clinical presentation of CHC is a white plaque that cannot be rubbed off and presenting most frequently in the commissural regions of the oral mucosa.

Treatment

Appropriate antifungal therapy usually leads to resolution of the condition and thus the lesion can be differentiated from oral leukoplakia of idiopathic origin.

Chronic hyperplastic candidosis/candidiasis is a variant of oral candidosis that typically presents as a white patch on the commissures of the oral mucosa. Clinically, the lesions are symptomless and regress after appropriate antifungal therapy and correction of underlying nutritional or other deficiencies. If the lesions are untreated, a minor proportion may demonstrate dysplasia and develop into carcinomas.

- Careful and routine follow-up observations of leukoplakia may be appropriate.
- Improved treatment outcomes may be realized with concomitant elimination of smoking, since this can often be a compromising factor.
- Topical application of clotrimazole mouthpaint three times a day over the lesion.
- These lesions respond to topical agents including imidazoles.
- When present in an immunocompromised person, such candidal lesions may require use of more toxic drugs such as amphotericin B.

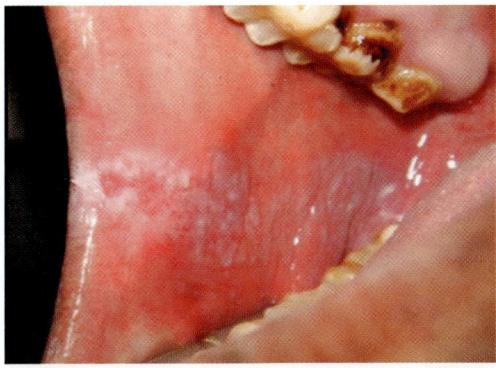

Fig. 5.30: A 39-year-old bidi smoker presented with an erythematous patch on the right buccal mucosa, surrounded by white patch extending from the retrocommissural region to posterior extent of buccal mucosa.

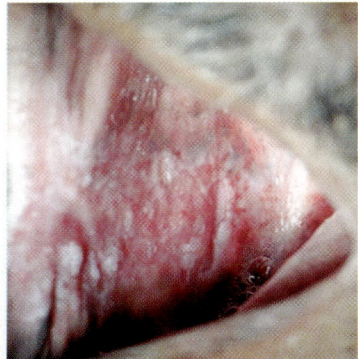

Fig. 5.31: A 45-year-old bidi smoker presented with a mixed red and white area on the entire right buccal mucosa.

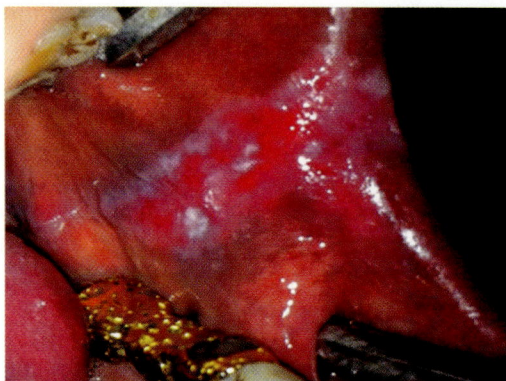

Fig. 5.32: Presence of a mixed erythematous and hyperkeratotic patch on the left buccal mucosa of a 45-year-old male patient, with a tobacco smoking habit.

Verrucous Leukoplakia

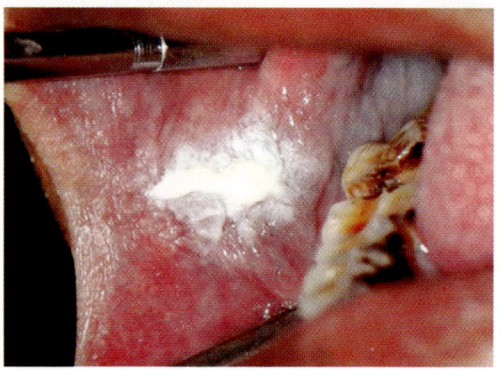

Fig. 5.33: Verrucous leukoplakia on the right buccal mucosa of a 40-year-old male patient with bidi and cigarette smoking habits.

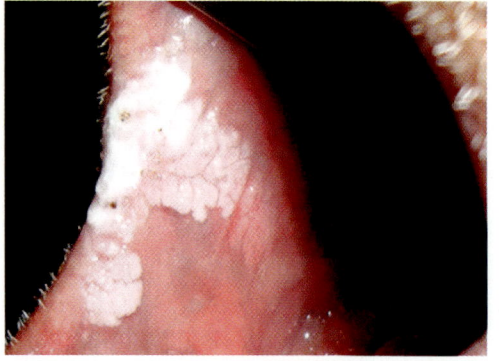

Fig. 5.34: A proliferative white patch on the right anterior region of buccal mucosa in a 56-year-old male bidi smoker.

Oral Submucous Fibrosis

Oral submucous fibrosis (OSF) is a chronic disorder characterized by fibrosis of the lining mucosa of the upper digestive tract involving the oral cavity, oropharynx, and frequently the upper third of the oesophagus, caused due to areca nut chewing habits.

The disease is characterized by the presence of palpable fibrous bands in the oral mucosa, ultimately leading to severe restriction of the movements of the mouth, including that of the tongue. On clinical examination, limitation of opening of the mouth may be obvious. In addition, the tongue may be small and exhibit very limited mobility and shows a marked loss of papillae.

The early and late forms of presentation are outlined in Table 5.1.

Table 5.1: Clinical presentations of oral submucous fibrosis

Early forms	Late presentation
Burning sensation, exacerbated by spicy food	Fibrous bands within mucosa
Vesiculation	Limitation of mouth opening
Blanching of mucosa	Narrowing of oropharyngeal orifice with distortion of uvula
Leathery mucosa	Woody changes to mucosa and tongue

Khanna JN and Andrade NN (1995) developed a group classification system for the surgical management of OSF.

- **Group I:** This is the earliest stage and is not associated with mouth opening limitations. It refers to patients with an interincisal distance of greater than 35 mm.

- **Group II:** This refers to patients with an interincisal distance of 26–35 mm.

- **Group III:** These are moderately advanced cases. This stage refers to patients with an interincisal distance of 15–26 mm. Fibrotic bands are visible at the soft palate, and pterygomandibular raphe and anterior pillars of fauces are present.

- **Group IVA:** Trismus is severe, with an interincisal distance of less than 15 mm and extensive fibrosis of all the oral mucosa.
- **Group IVB:** Disease is most advanced, with premalignant and malignant changes throughout the mucosa.

Treatment

Currently, intralesional steroids are the main treatment modality. These are injected into the fibrotic bands weekly for 6–8 weeks with regular monitoring of mouth opening. Patients are advised to do mouth-opening exercises, for example, by placing ice cream sticks in their mouth and gradually increasing the number. Hyaluronidase, which facilitates the breakdown of connective tissue, can be combined with the steroids (dexamethasone) for injection. The list of other treatment modalities is extensive and includes use of micronutrients and minerals, carbon dioxide laser, pentoxifylline, lycopene, immunized milk, interferon gamma, turmeric, hyalase, chymotrypsin and collagenase. Surgical modalities like surgical excision of bands, coronoidectomy, myotomy have been tried.

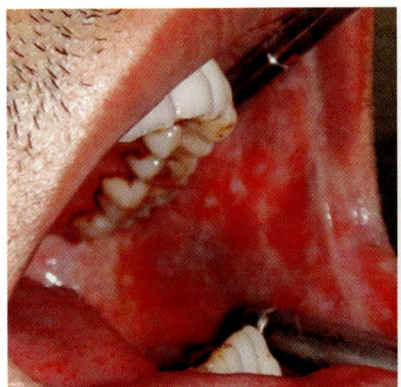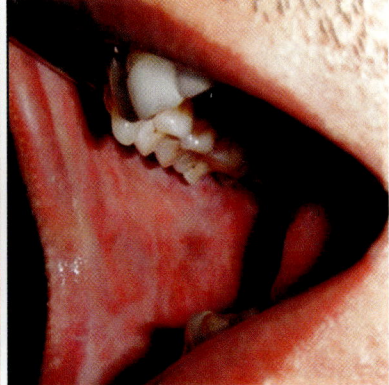

Fig. 5.35: Atrophy of left buccal mucosa and blanching of right buccal mucosa in a 30-year-old male patient with oral submucous fibrosis.

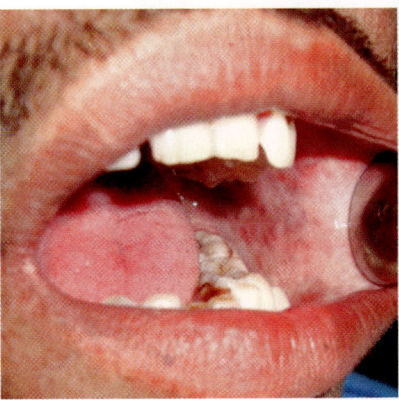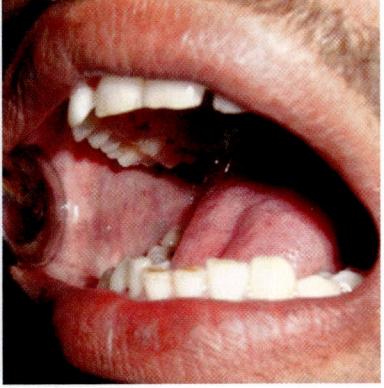

Fig. 5.36: Reduced mouth opening with a characteristic marble-like appearance of buccal mucosae in a young patient with oral submucous fibrosis.

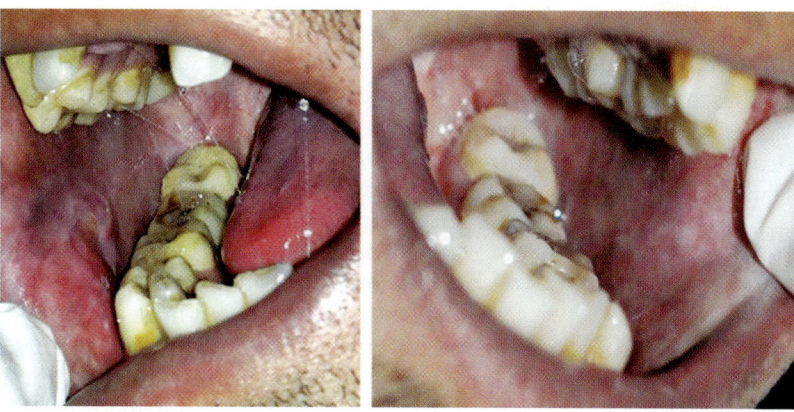

Fig. 5.37: A 25-year-old male with gutkha chewing habit presented with reduced mouth opening and blanched buccal mucosae with palpable fibrous bands.

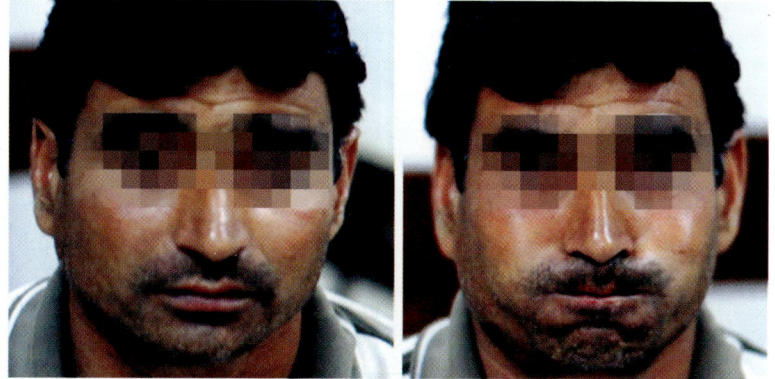

Fig. 5.38: Inability to blow cheeks in a 38-year-old male with oral submucous fibrosis. The patient had a combination of gutkha and tobacco chewing; cigarette smoking and alcohol consumption habits.

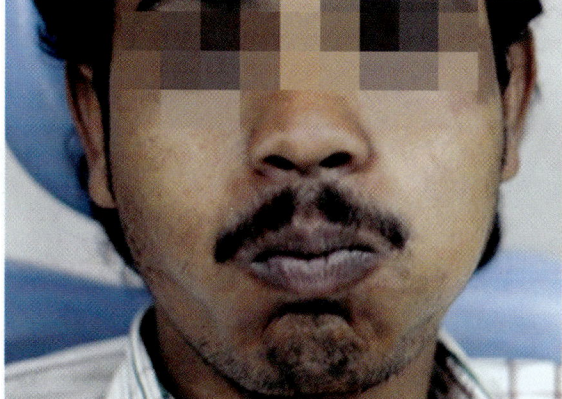

Fig. 5.39: A 25-year-old male with gutkha chewing habit presented with unilateral oral submucous fibrosis. On blowing, fullness of cheek was observed on left side only.

Carcinoma

The most important of oral mucosal lesion is the carcinoma, in most cases, a squamous cell carcinoma, because it may cause death if not treated at an early stage. The location of an oral carcinoma is often associated with various smoking and/or chewing habits involving tobacco and/or areca (betel) nut.

Oral cancer prevalence has decreased from the mid-1960s until the latest (2004) National Cancer Institute Survey. In 2004, approximately 157,000 (0.11% of) men and 87,000 (0.07% of) women had oral cancer.

Clinical Presentation

The carcinoma may develop in a white patch (an area of leukoplakia) or in a red area (an erythroplakia) but many carcinomas arise in an area of mucosa that previously appeared normal. The appearance of the surface of the tumor is very variable; it may be relatively smooth and white or red, but commonly the surface is nodular or ulcerated and the ulcer may have a raised rolled margin. In the later stages there may be a soft fungating mass that bleeds readily. If the carcinoma arises on lip, where the surface can become dry, there is often a crusted or scaly appearance or the surface can appear warty. The verrucous carcinoma is a predominantly exophytic growth, and presents as a painless warty mass that usually has a white nodular surface. Despite the serious nature of the lesion, there may be a little or no pain.

Except in some early and small lesions, there is usually induration—the tissue feels firm and thickened—either throughout the lesion, or at the margins if there is ulceration. Where the tumor occurs on a mobile part of the mucosa, there may be fixation and loss of mobility because the tumor has involved deeper tissues.

Treatment

The diagnosis is confirmed by computed tomography or magnetic resonance imaging along with biopsy and a standardized histopathological examination. Advanced disease (stages T3 and T4) should be treated by surgery followed by radiotherapy, with or without chemotherapy. 20% of the patients overall go on to have a recurrence, usually within 2 to 3 years of the initial treatment. The 5-year survival rate is somewhat above 50%.

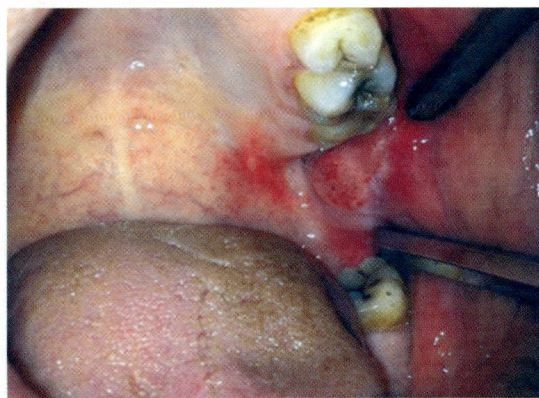

Fig. 5.40: A 58-year-old male patient with tobacco chewing habit presented with an erythematous ulcer surrounded by a white margin on the upper left buccal mucosa, posterior to the third molar tooth. An incisional biopsy of the ulcer revealed moderately differentiated squamous cell carcinoma.

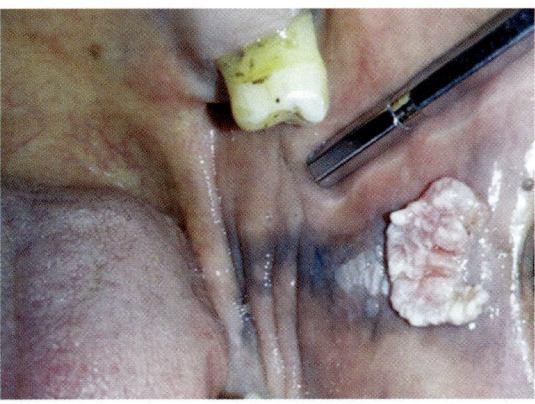

Fig. 5.41: A 59-year-old bidi smoker presented with a proliferative growth on the left buccal mucosa, histopathologically diagnosed as squamous cell carcinoma.

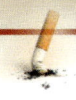

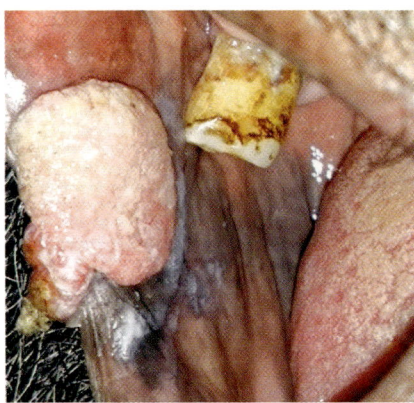

Fig. 5.42: Presence of a raised smooth surfaced growth on the right anterior buccal mucosa, surrounded by a faint leukoplakia.

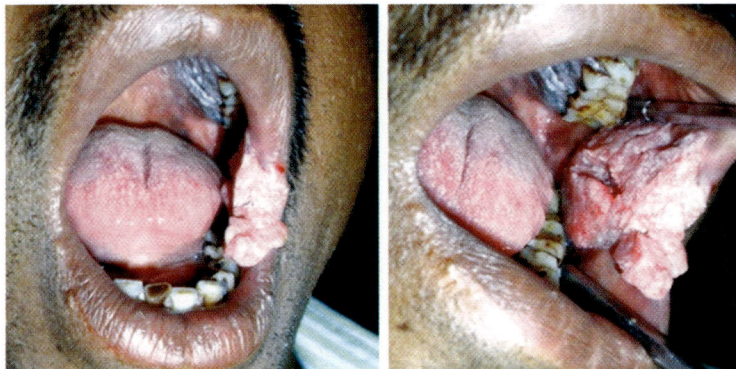

Fig. 5.43: An exophytic growth seen on the left commissural region, extending up to the posterior region of buccal mucosa in a 50-year-old male with tobacco chewing habit.

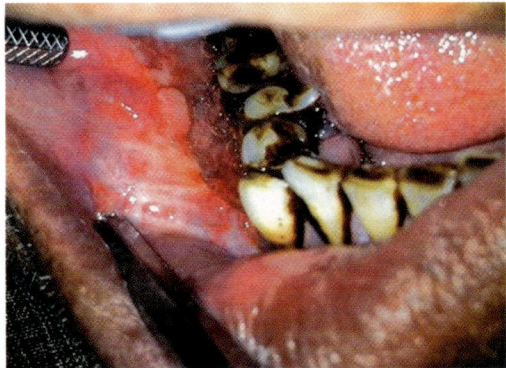

Fig. 5.44: A 52-year-old male pan chewer with oral submucous fibrosis, presented with an ulcer with a granulomatous base on the gingivo-bucco-vestibular fold since 6 months. Histopathology report revealed a well-differentiated squamous cell carcinoma.

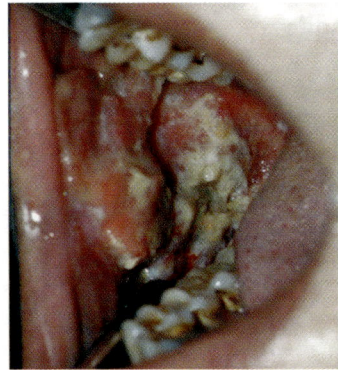

Fig. 5.45: A 40-year-old female patient with pan chewing habit presented with an ulceroproliferative growth on the right buccal mucosa that was exquisitely tender to palpation and bled readily on slight provocation.

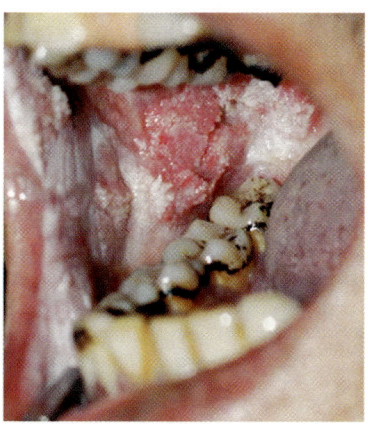

Fig. 5.46: Ulceroproliferative growth on right buccal mucosa secondary to pan chewing habit in a 39-year-old male.

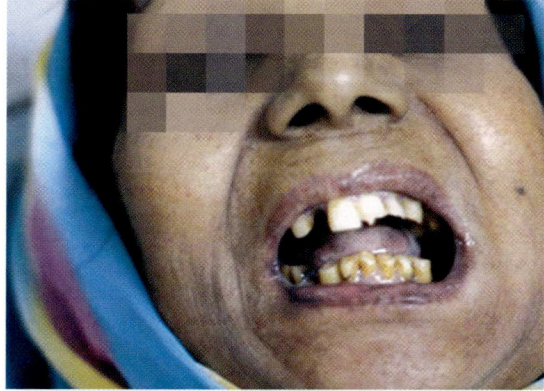

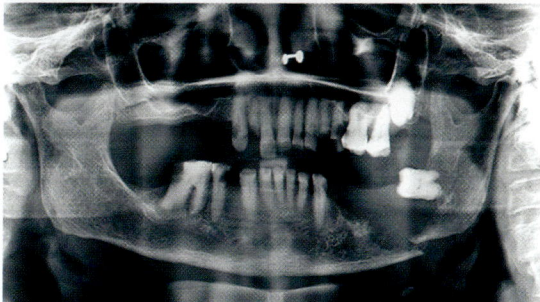

Fig. 5.47: A 50-year-old female with tobacco chewing habit presented with oral submucous fibrosis (restricted mouth opening and palpable fibrous bands) and a non-healing, painful ulcer on the left buccal mucosa. A panoramic radiograph revealed bone resorption and pathological fracture of the left lower border of mandible.

LABIAL MUCOSA

Chemical Burn

The habit of placement of tobacco and slaked lime in the labial mucosa/vestibular region will produce a thin white scrapable film, due to the alkaline nature of slaked lime. The thin film can be easily removed to expose an underlying erythematous area. There may be formation of ulcers and a burning or painful sensation at the site.

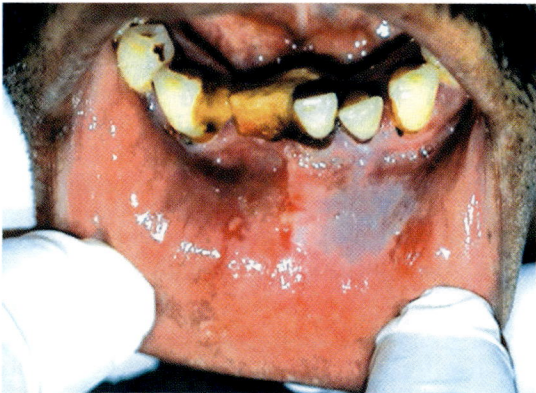

Fig. 5.48: Chemical burn with ulceration on the lower labial mucosa in a 46-year-old male patient with the habit of chewing tobacco and slaked lime.

Frictional Keratosis

Frictional/focal keratosis is a white lesion related to chronic rubbing or friction against an oral mucosal surface; resulting in the formation of a presumably protective layer, analogous to callus of skin. It may also appear on varied sites in non-tobacco users, due to other causative factors like sharp tooth, chronic cheek or lip biting. A positive history of tobacco-consumption and absence of any other factors of mechanical trauma will aid in the identification of cause.

Clinical Features

It presents as a white patch on the site adjacent to the causative factor (sharp tooth, or other foreign bodies).

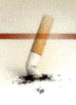

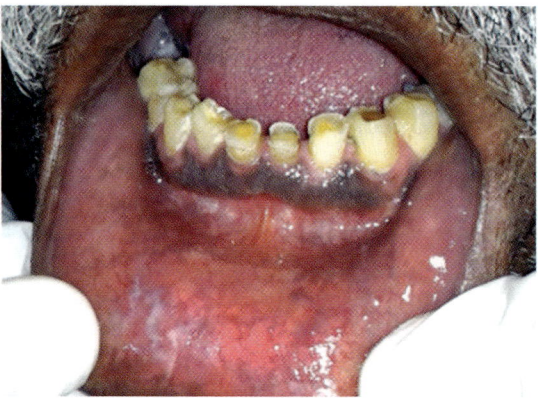

Fig. 5.49: Frictional keratosis seen on the right side of lower labial mucosa due to sharp incisal edges of mandibular anterior teeth, associated with tobacco chewing.

Treatment

Gradual regression of mild lesions is possible if the causal factors are eliminated.

Chewer's Mucosa

The habit of pan chewing, usually, results in peeling of the epithelium, forming tissue tags and provides an orange-pink color to the mucosa. It is commonly visible at the site of placement of the quid. The buccal mucosa is most frequently affected, and has a prevalence of 0.2%. Differential diagnoses include cheek

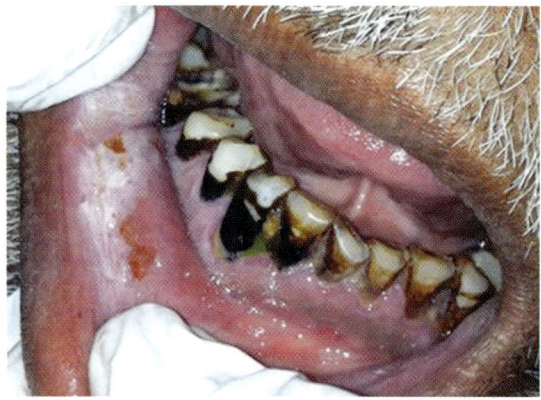

Fig. 5.50: A white patch with a red-orange colored patch right labial mucosa, associated with pan chewing.

biting, with which it has a number of similarities, and other predominantly white lesions that may have taken up stains from tobacco and other substances.

Leukoplakia

Leukoplakia of the lip is rare and usually limited to the labial mucosa, without infringing upon the vermilion border.

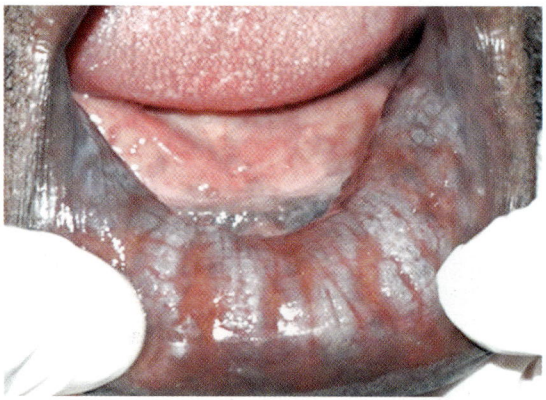

Fig. 5.51: Presence of a milder form of homogenous leukoplakia on lower labial mucosa in a bidi smoker.

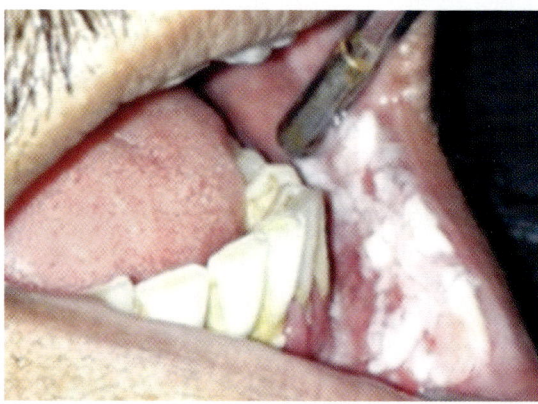

Fig. 5.52: Verrucous leukoplakia on left labial mucosa in a 53-year-old male with bidi and cigarette smoking habits.

Oral Submucous Fibrosis

In oral submucous fibrosis, the labial mucosae show blanching in early cases and development of palpable fibrous bands around rima oris.

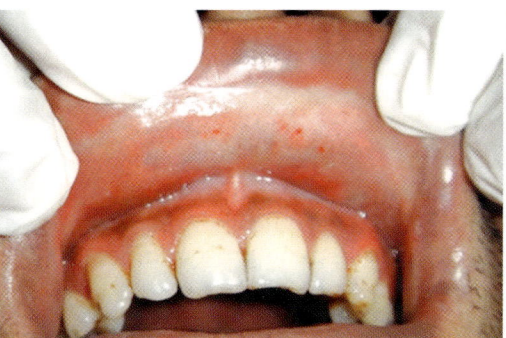
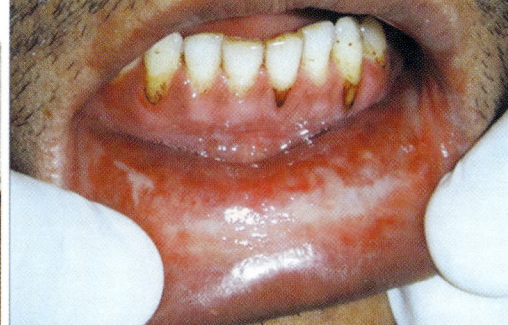

Fig. 5.53: Blanching of upper and lower labial mucosae seen in a patient with oral submucous fibrosis.

VESTIBULE

Chemical Burn

Chemical burn results from topical application of irritating substances, especially slaked lime. Placement of slaked lime in combination with tobacco in the vestibular region is commonly a causative agent. Similar lesion is observed with analgesic tablets.

Clinical Presentation

The lesion consists of a slough that is produced by the coagulation of protein in the superficial epithelial cells. There is desquamation of the epithelium and possible ulcer formation at the site of placement.

Treatment

Discontinuation of the habit will reverse the condition steadily.

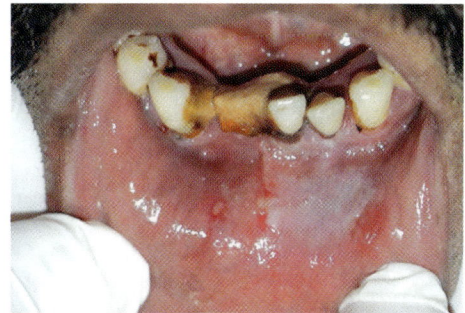

Fig. 5.55: Chemical burn caused due to use of slaked lime and tobacco in the right labial vestibule region.

Tobacco Pouch Keratosis

Placement of smokeless tobacco in the labial and buccal vestibule is a common practice. It gives rise to leukoplakia-like manifestations of those areas of the mucosa that come in contact with the tobacco quid.

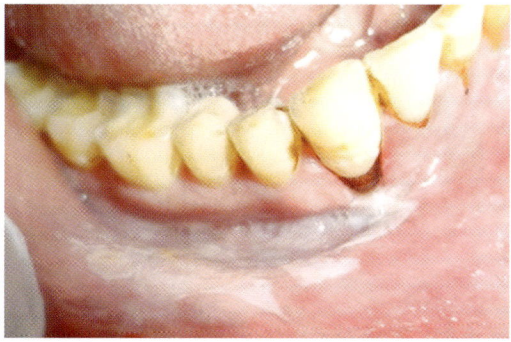

Fig. 5.54: Presence of chemical burn in the buccal vestibule in a 38-year-old user of tobacco and slaked lime.

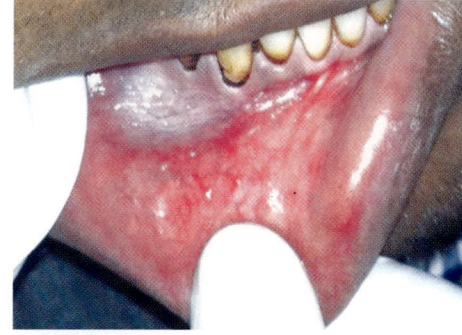

Fig. 5.56: A 26-year-old male with habit of using tobacco presented with a corrugated white patch on the right side of labial vestibule.

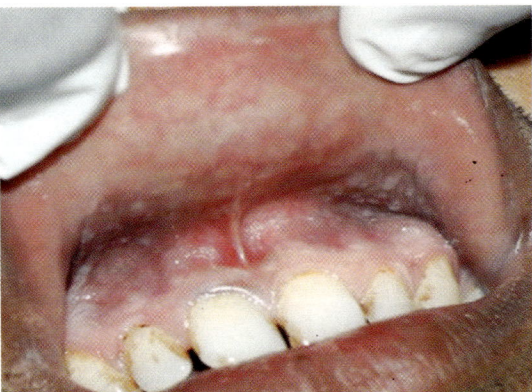

Fig. 5.57: Tobacco pouch keratosis in a 24-year-old male patient with habit of chewing tobacco.

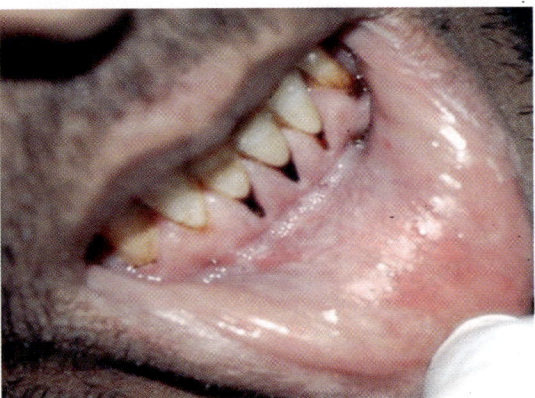

Fig. 5.58: Mild degree of keratosis seen in the lower labial vestibular region associated with tobacco preparation in a 29-year-old male.

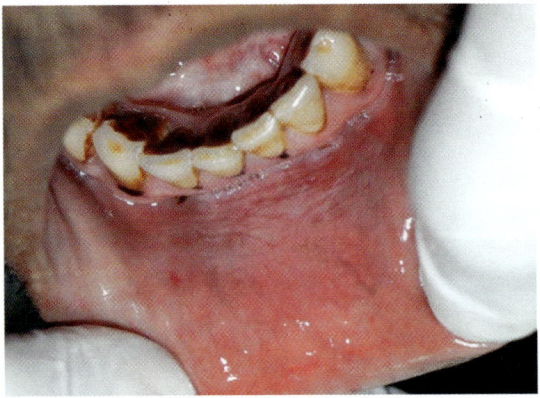

Fig. 5.59: Tobacco pouch keratosis with attrition of mandibular anterior teeth associated with placement of tobacco in this region.

Pan Stains

This type of lesion is seen in association with placement of pan in the vestibule.

Clinical Presentation

It appears as a red discoloration of the oral mucosa in betel quid chewers. The underlying areas may assume a pseudomembranous or wrinkled appearance.

Treatment

Refraining from the habit and regular rinsing usually clears the stain.

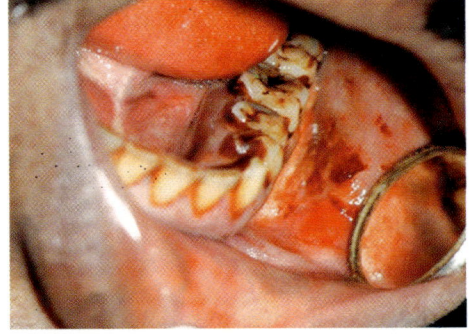

Fig. 5.60: A 55-year-old pan chewer presented with pan stains on the left buccal vestibule region.

Leukoplakia

A leukoplakic patch may be seen in the vestibule, i.e. one of the sites of placement of tobacco, which is well demarcated and non-scrapable.

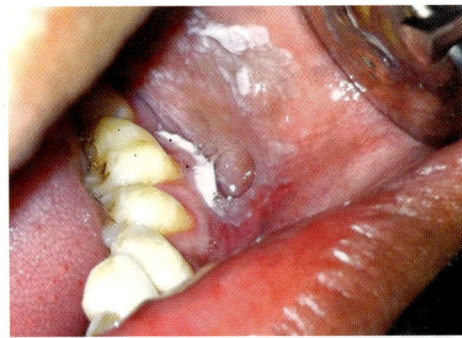

Fig. 5.61: A white patch on the left buccal mucosa and vestibular region, non-scrapable associated with tobacco chewing habit.

Carcinoma

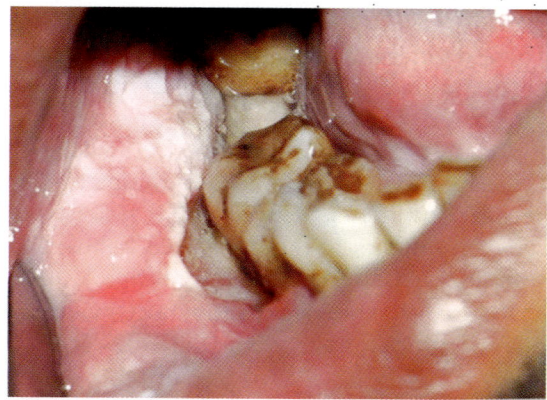

Fig. 5.62: An ulcer on the right lower buccal vestibule with undermined edges, with a surrounding leukoplakia. The patient was a gutkha chewer.

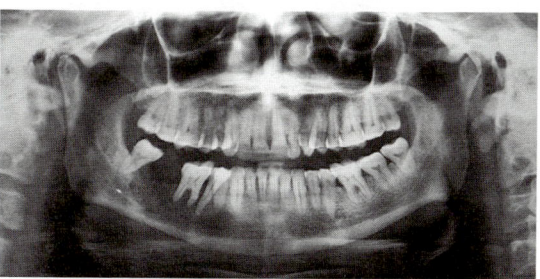

Fig. 5.63: An orthopantomogram of the same patient reveals severe bone destruction in the right posterior mandible, giving rise to a floating teeth appearance i.r.t. 45, 46, 47.

ANGLE OF MOUTH

Angular Cheilitis

Angular cheilitis is an inflammatory condition that occurs in one or both angles of the mouth. It refers to the development of erythematous, scaling fissures at the corners of the mouth. Facial wrinkling at the corners of the mouth and along the nasolabial fold especially in older people leads to a chronically moist environment that predisposes to this lesion. This wrinkling is worse in long-term denture wearers because there is resorption of bone on which the dentures rest leading to a

reduction in height of the lower face when the mouth is closed. Other factors implicated in the etiology of this condition are iron deficiency anemia and vitamin B_{12} deficiency.

Clinical Presentation

This condition typically presents with erythema, painful cracking, scaling, bleeding, and ulceration at the corners of the mouth.

Treatment

Addressing the underlying cause with use of topical antifungal paints will treat the condition.

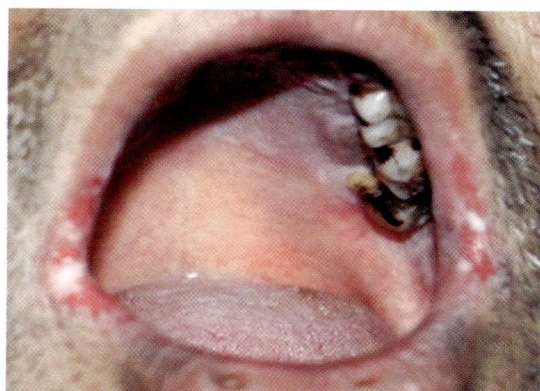

Fig. 5.64: A 45-year-old male smoker presented with the presence of an erythematous area on the angle of mouth bilaterally associated with bidi smoker.

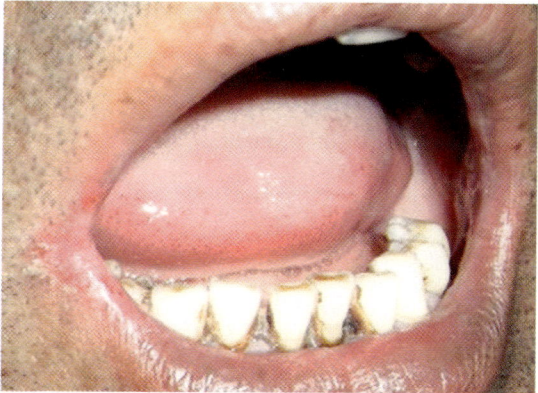

Fig. 5.65: Presence of an non-scrapable erythematous area on the angle of mouth on the right side of angle of mouth in a 46-year-old male with bidi smoking habit.

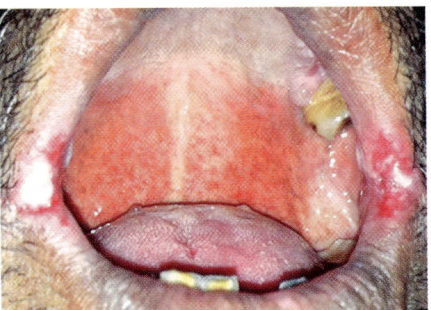

Fig. 5.66: Angular cheilitis bilaterally on corner of mouth in a 50-year-old smoker.

Leukoplakia

The lip is an uncommon site for development of leukoplakia. It may be seen as a continuation of the leukoplakic patch present on the buccal mucosa. It usually does not involve the vermilion border, as opposed to carcinoma.

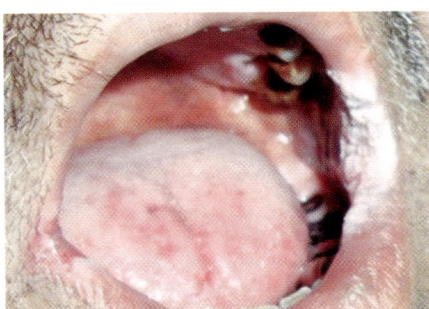

Fig. 5.67: Homogenous leukoplakia on the left side and angular cheilitis on the right side angle of mouth in a 51-year-old bidi smoker.

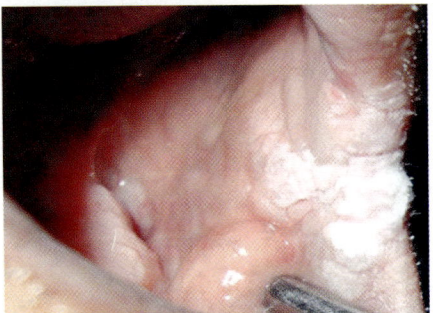

Fig. 5.68: Verrucous leukoplakia on the left commissural region with a cracked mud appearance, non-scrapable, associated with bidi smoking habit in a 62-year-old male.

GINGIVA AND ALVEOLAR RIDGE

Irritation Fibroma

These proliferations are painless pedunculated or sessile masses in different colors, from light pink to red. The surface appearance is variable from non-ulcerated smooth to ulcerated mass. Lesion size varies from a few millimeters to several centimeters. Such similar lesions are seen in patients without tobacco habits; the source of irritation being different.

Figure 5.70 shows a postoperative view, at one-month follow up of the patient.

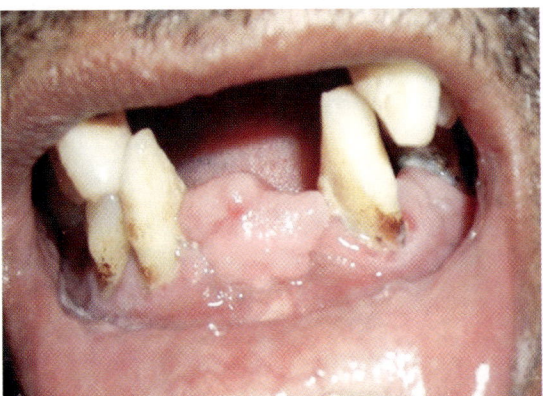

Fig. 5.69: A 45-year-old male patient, with a habit of smoking bidi since 20 years, reported with a non-tender, firm and pedunculated growth on the mandibular anterior region of gingiva since a month. Histopathological examination revealed fibroepithelial hyperplasia with abnormal keratinization.

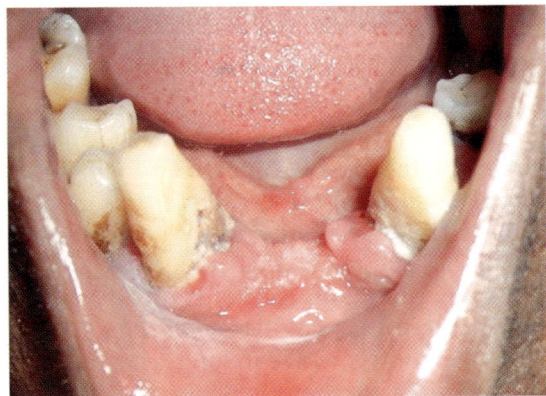

Fig. 5.70: Postoperative view of the same patient.

Erythematous Candidiasis

Fungal infections in humans occur as a result of defects in the immune system. An increasing emergence in oral Candidal and non-Candidal fungal infections is evident in the past decade owing to the rise in the immunodeficient and immunocompromised population globally. Oral Candidal infection usually involves a compromised host and the compromise may be local or systemic.

Inflammatory lesions of the mucosa beneath the maxillary dentures are known as denture stomatitis. It is commonly seen in denture wearers and smokers.

Clinical Presentation

Erythematous candidiasis clinically presents as localized erythema of the oral mucosa with or without associated symptoms.

Treatment

Cessation of deleterious habits and evading other underlying causes is foremost. The lesion responds well to anti-fungal agents.

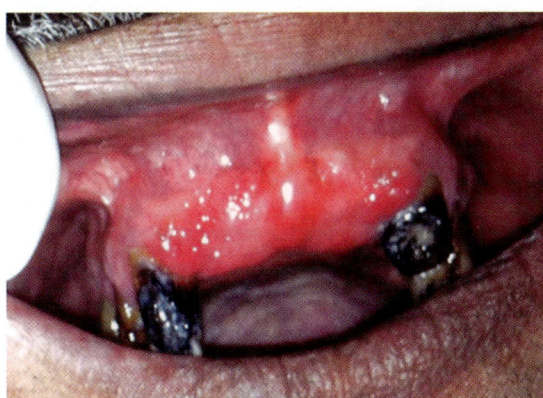

Fig. 5.71: Presence of diffused erythema on the maxillary anterior gingiva associated with removable prosthesis in a 52-year-old bidi smoker.

Leukoplakia

Localization of leukoplakia on the gingiva, adjacent vestibulum with its mobile alveolar mucosa is less common. For verrucous leuko-plakia, the mandibular gingiva is a common site.

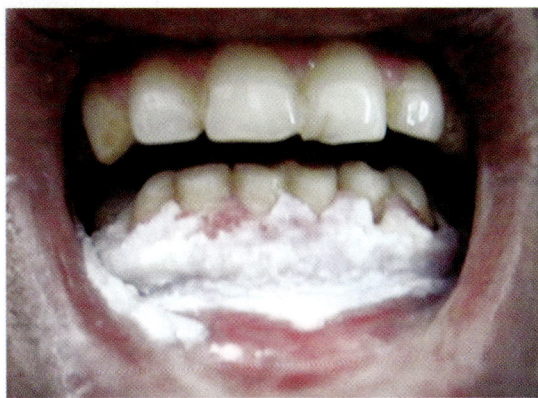

Fig. 5.72: Presence of a white colored verrucous growth on the mandibular anterior gingiva and labial vestibule, with multiple projections extending into the interdental spaces, associated with tobacco chewing.

Carcinoma

Gingival carcinoma occurs three times more commonly on the mandibular gingiva than maxilla. In dentulous patients, the gingiva carcinoma is easy to misinterpret as the clinical signs are similar to those of odontogenic infections and periodontitis.

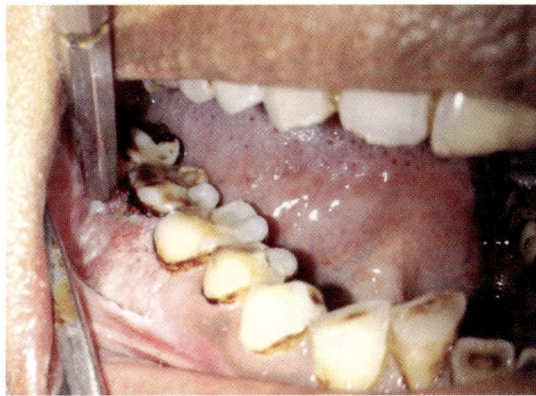

Fig. 5.73: A proliferative growth with minute papillary projections associated with free and attached gingiva of mandibular left first and second molar teeth, in a tobacco chewer.

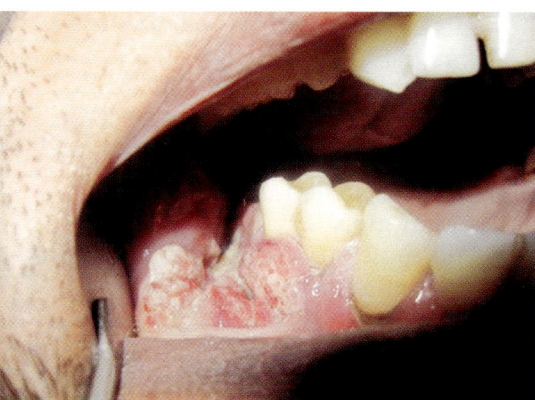

Fig. 5.74: Presence of a breach in the mandibular posterior gingiva and underlying alveolar bone, attached to a pale yellow proliferative growth, interspersed with pin-point erythematous areas, with the growth dipping into buccal vestibule. The patient was a tobacco chewer and bidi smoker.

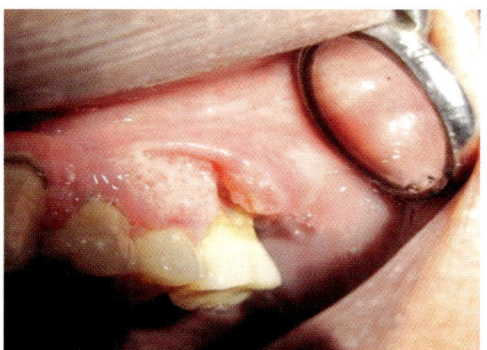 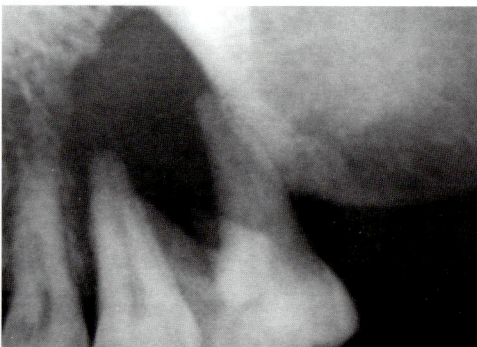

Fig. 5.75: An ulceroproliferative growth seen on the posterior region of buccal aspect of gingiva in a 47-year-old tobacco chewer. The ulcer appears to be white in color, bounded on one side by a rolled border that is thickened in the posterior region. An intra-oral periapical radiograph shows localized triangular area of bone loss, i.e. hanging-drop appearance, around the apices of maxillary left second premolar and first molar teeth.

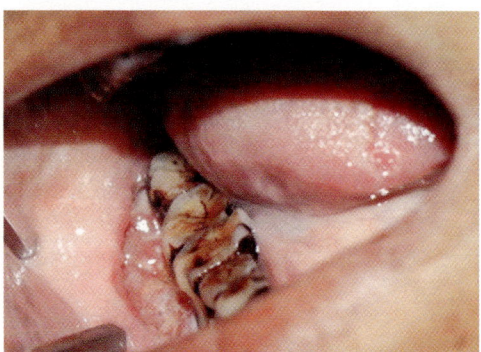 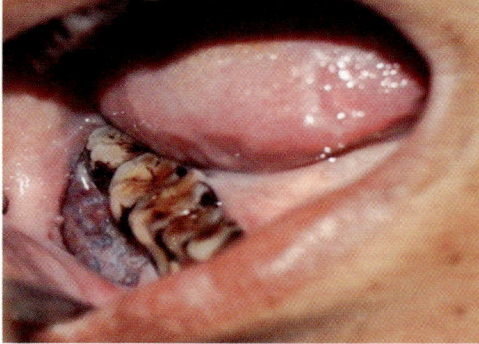

Fig. 5.76: An ill-defined shallow ulcer on the mandibular right posterior gingiva and buccal vestibule with an erythematous area, in a 53-year-old female with tobacco chewing habit. The ulcer had sharp boundaries and appeared indurated on palpation. The ulcer retained toluidine blue stain.

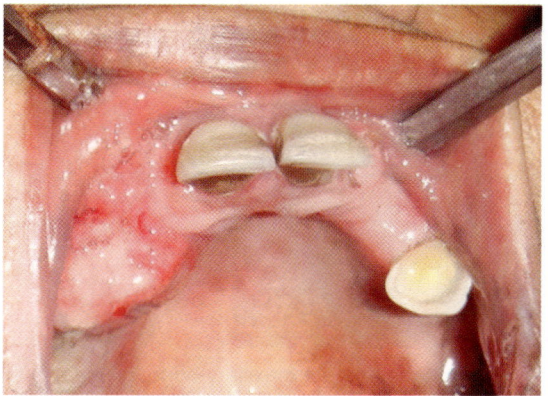

Fig. 5.77: An ill-defined growth on the maxillary right anterior alveolar ridge region, i.e. at the site of the maxillary right lateral incisor and canine. The growth is pale-pink with a few erythematous areas, and hard on palpation.

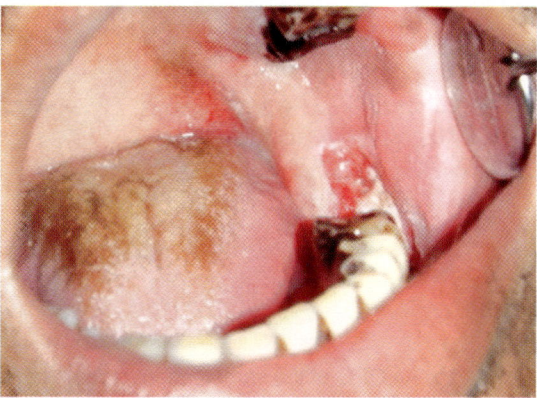

Fig. 5.79: A tobacco chewer had a non-healing ulcer on the left mandibular ridge. The ulcer was erythematous, had rolled borders, and indurated on palpation.

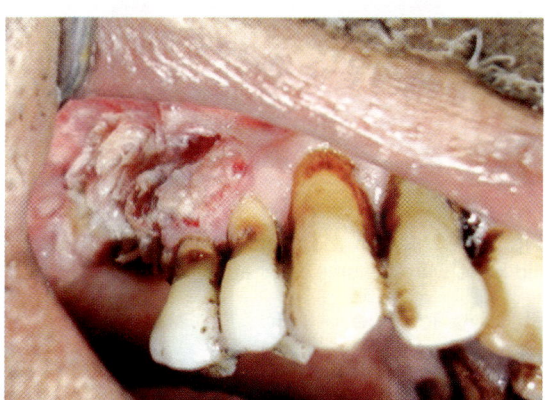

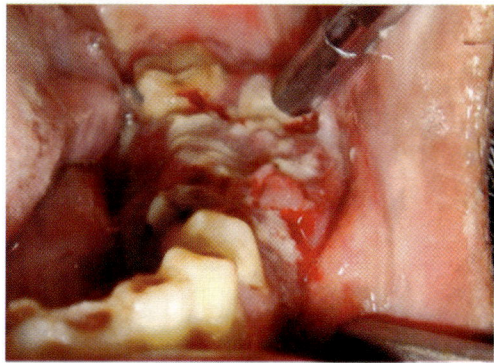

Fig. 5.80: An ulcer on the mandibular left alveolar ridge in a gutkha chewer, with everted margins and was covered with a dirty-white surface, and tendency to bleed on slight provocation.

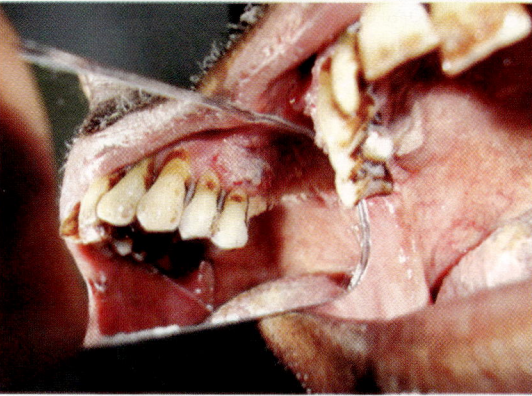

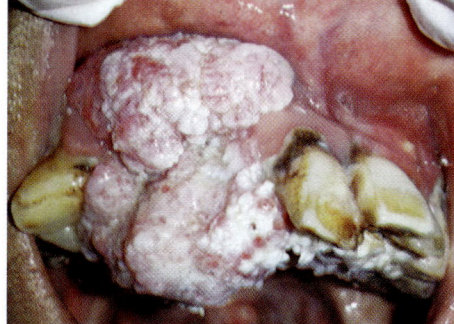

Fig. 5.78: A dirty-white verrucous growth on the maxillary right posterior aspect of gingiva, extending from the buccal vestibule to the palate.

Fig. 5.81a: A white-colored verrucous growth on the anterior maxillary gingival and alveolar ridge in a 69-year-old female with pan and plain areca nut chewing habits.

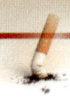

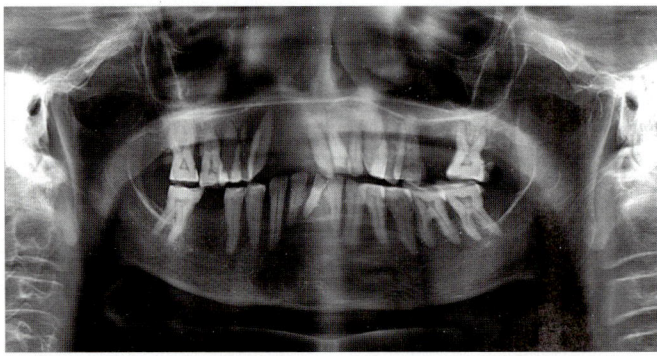

Fig. 5.81b: An OPG of the same patient reveals bone destruction in the anterior maxillary bone, giving rise to a floating tooth appearance i.r.t. 13.

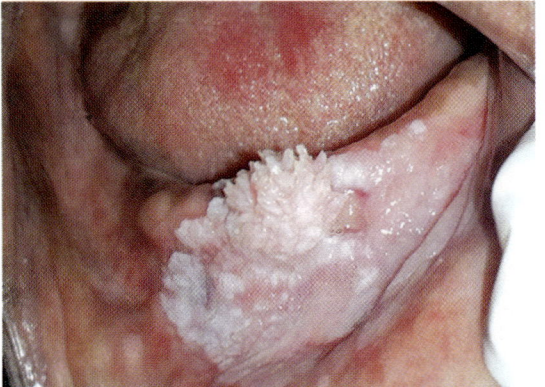

Fig. 5.82: A white verrucous growth on the mandibular anterior alveolar ridge, in a 70-year-old male bidi smoker.

TONGUE

Median Rhomboid Glossitis

Median rhomboid glossitis (MRG) is an uncommon benign abnormality of the tongue, most frequently affecting men. It is typically located around the midline of the dorsum of the tongue, anterior to the lingual "V", appearing as a reddish, rhomboid area, depapillated, flat maculate or mamillated and raised by 2–5 mm. It is now thought to be a form of candidiasis, also known as central papillary atrophy and posterior midline atrophic candidiasis. It occurs in as many as 1% of adults. This condition was once thought to represent a developmental defect.

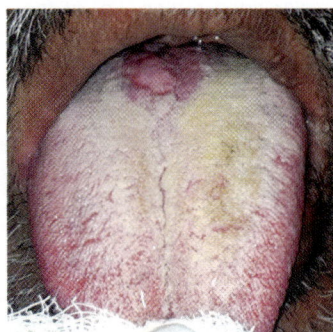

Fig. 5.83: Median rhomboid glossitis in a 65-year-old male with bidi smoking habit.

Stained Tongue

Pan chewers may develop orange-red stains on the dorsum of tongue, due to leaching out of the colors of various components of pan. The stains usually are cleared on scrubbing regularly and discontinuation of the habit.

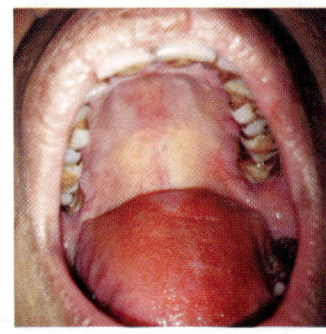

Fig. 5.84: Pan stains with median rhomboid glossitis in a 47-year-old male patient with pan chewing habit.

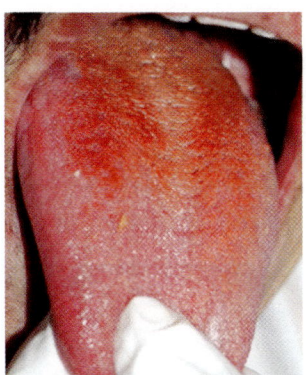

Fig. 5.85: A 35-year-old male with pan and zarda chewing habits presented with yello-orange stains on the postero-dorsal aspect of tongue.

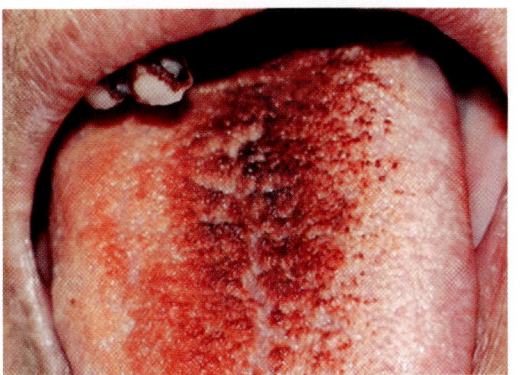

Fig. 5.86: Orange to brown stains on the dorsal aspect of tongue in a 50-year-old male with pan chewing habit.

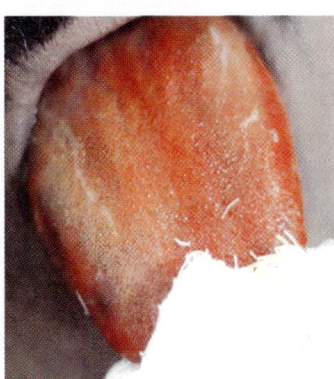

Fig. 5.87: A 45-year-old male presented with an orange-red stained tongue associated with pan chewing habit.

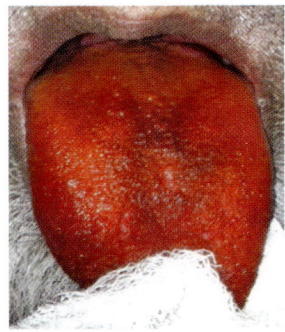

Fig. 5.88: Pan stained tongue in a 70-year-old male pan chewer.

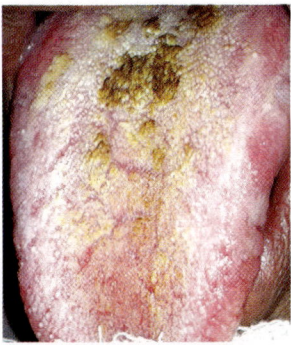

Fig. 5.89: Coated tongue in a 66-year-old bidi smoker and tobacco chewer.

Irritation Fibroma

Irritation fibroma is a form of reactive hyperplasias. The lesion must be distinguished from that caused by tobacco, by identifying the source of irritation. Within the mouth, buccal, labial and lateral tongue sites account for the most common sites.

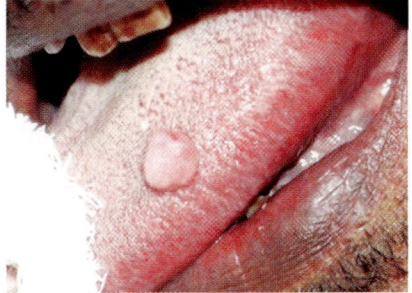

Fig. 5.90: Presence of a pale pink soft tissue growth on the left side of dorsum of tongue in a 46-year-old male patient with tobacco chewing habit.

Lichenoid Reaction

The lesion generally presents at the site of placement of quid. The most frequent location is the buccal mucosa, gingiva and tongue. Other causes of lichenoid reaction like drugs, dental materials must be identified.

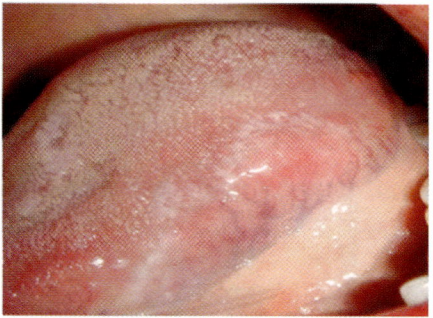

Fig. 5.91: Lichenoid reaction on left lateral border of tongue in a 35-year-old female patient with tobacco chewing habit.

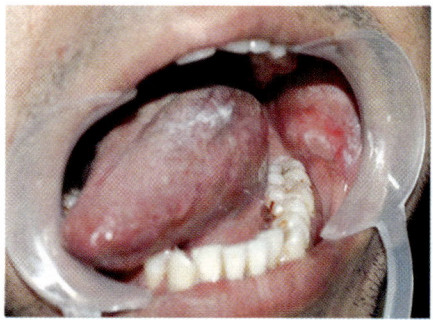

Fig. 5.92: Lichenoid reaction on dorsal surface on the tongue and the left buccal mucosa associated with tobacco chewing.

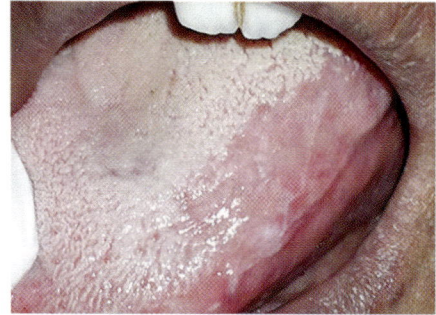

Fig. 5.93: Lichenoid reaction on left dorsum and lateral border of tongue in a 29-year-old pan masala chewer.

Leukoplakia

Lingual leukoplakia is localized on the lateral borders of tongue, the dorsum and ventral surface of tongue. Malignant transformation of leukoplakia on the lingual borders and on the ventral surface as well as floor of mouth occurs more frequently than in other regions.

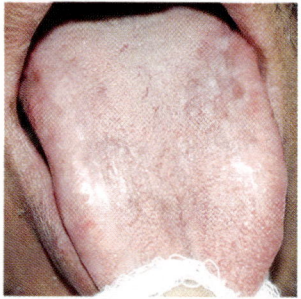

Fig. 5.94: Presence of a white patch on the left side of dorsum of tongue in a 25-year-old male with bidi smoking, tobacco chewing and alcohol consumption habits.

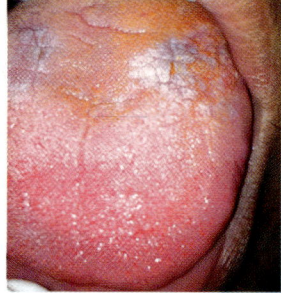

Fig. 5.95: Homogenous leukoplakia on the dorsal aspect of tongue with pan stains associated with betel quid chewing in a 45-year-old male.

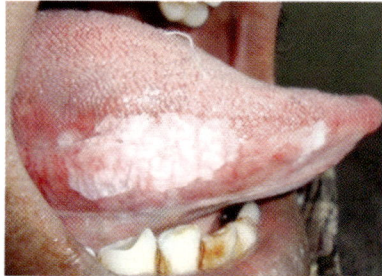

Fig. 5.96: A 48-year-old male presented with a white non-scrapable patch, with a cracked mud appearance on the right lateral border of tongue, associated with bidi smoking and tobacco chewing habits.

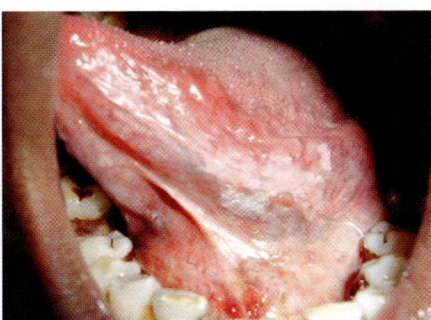

Fig. 5.97: Homogenous leukoplakia on the left lateral border of tongue in a 38-year-old male with bidi smoking habit.

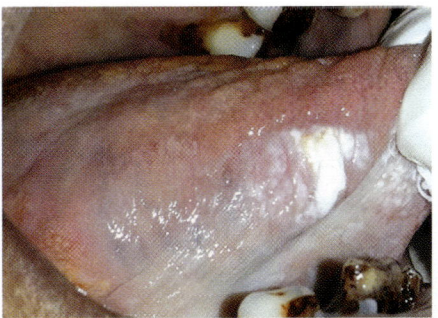

Fig. 5.98: A small thick white patch on the right ventral surface of tongue in a 46-year-old male with bidi smoking habit.

Oral Submucous Fibrosis

Oral submucous fibrosis may lead to blanching of the mucosa on ventral surface of tongue, in early cases, and difficulty in tongue movements in advanced stages.

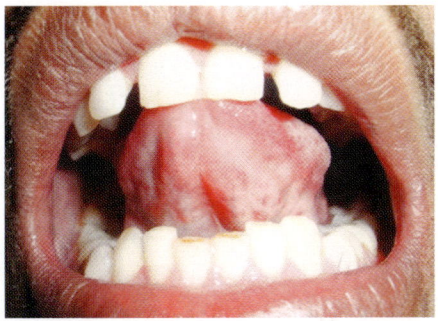

Fig. 5.99: Blanching and incomplete protrusion of tongue in a young patient with oral submucous fibrosis caused due to gutkha chewing habit.

Carcinoma

Carcinoma of the tongue is usually exophytic, in conjunction with ulcerations of varying depths. The ulcers must be distinguished from those that are traumatic in nature. The lesion is surrounded by leukoplakia in some cases.

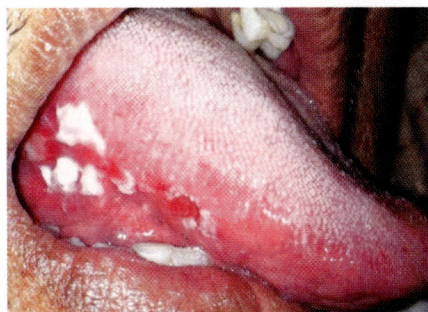

Fig. 5.100: Carcinoma on right lateral border of tongue presenting as a mixed red and white patch, in a patient with gutkha chewing habit.

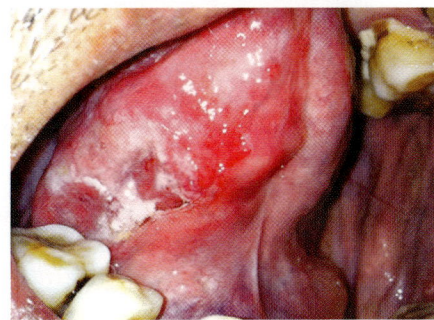

Fig. 5.101: Carcinoma on right lateral border of tongue in a 60-year-old male patient with tobacco chewing habit.

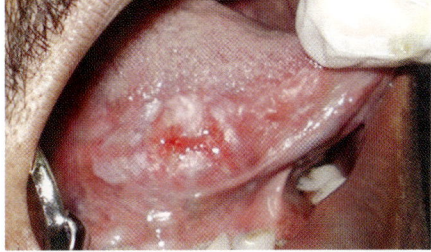

Fig. 5.102: Presence of a predominantly white and red patch on the right lateral border of tongue, non-scrapable, painful and tender on palpation in a 56-year-old male patient with bidi smoking and tobacco chewing habits.

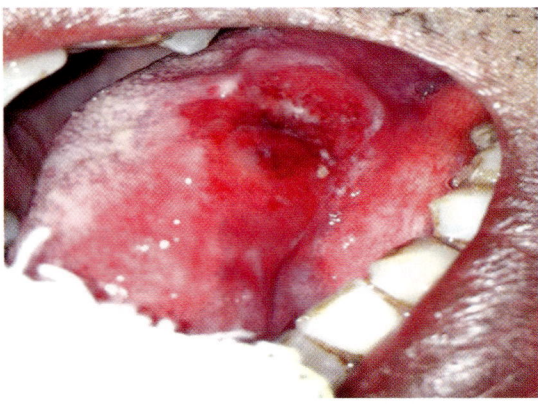

Fig. 5.103: A 51-year-old male with tobacco chewing habit presented with a deep indurated ulcer on left lateral border of tongue with bleeding tendency.

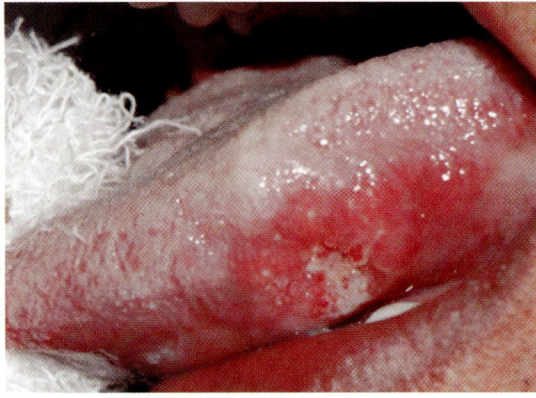

Fig. 5.104: A 36-year-old male with pan masala chewing habit presented with an ulcer, which had indurated floor and raised edges; on the left lateral border of tongue.

FLOOR OF MOUTH

Leukoplakia

The most common site for leukoplakia with severe dysplasia and invasive carcinoma is the lateral aspect of the tongue, the floor of the mouth, and the gums. It is, therefore, essential to include these sites in the clinical examination to aid early diagnosis. It is also important to monitor leukoplakias without dysplastic features as they can occasionally be the site of carcinoma.

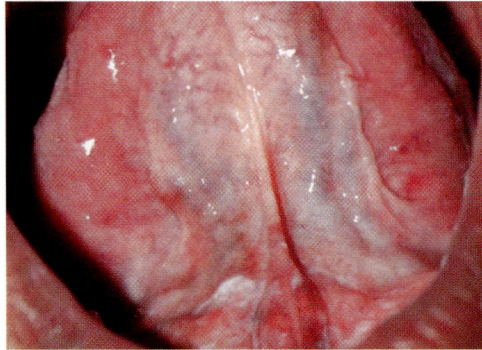

Fig. 5.105: Presence of a small homogenous white patch on the floor of mouth in a 56-year-old male smoker.

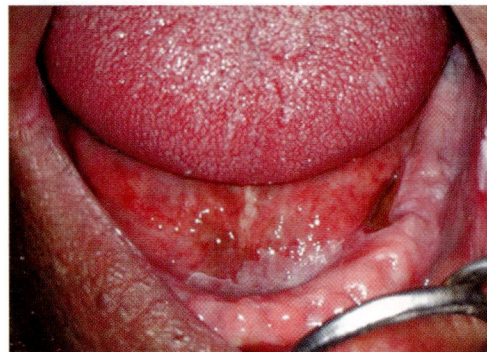

Fig. 5.106: Presence of a thin white patch on the floor of mouth in a 67-year-old bidi smoker.

Oral Submucous Fibrosis

On floor of mouth, blanching and a typical marble-like appearance is observed in oral submucous fibrosis.

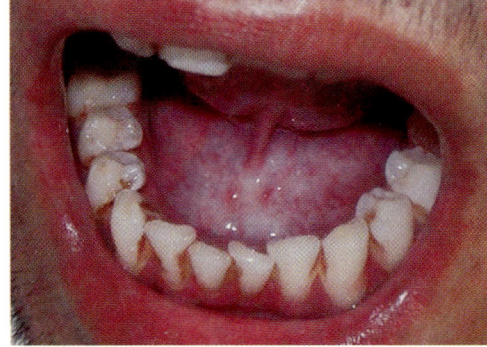

Fig. 5.107: Blanching of floor of mouth in a young patient with oral submucous fibrosis, due to areca nut chewing habit.

PALATE

Fibroma

It represents fibrous hyperplasia caused due to chronic irritation. Tobacco chewing could give rise to a fibroma. Other causes of chronic irritation such as maxillary denture must be identified. It occurs on the gingiva, buccal mucosa, lips, tongue, and palate.

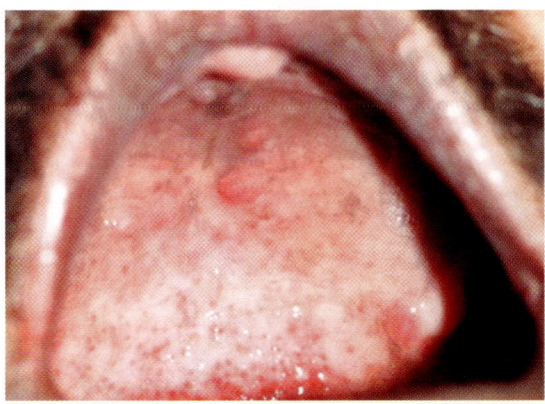

Fig. 5.108: A 53-year-old bidi smoker presented with a pale pink, slightly raised, well circumscribed, sessile soft tissue growth on the anterior one-third of palate.

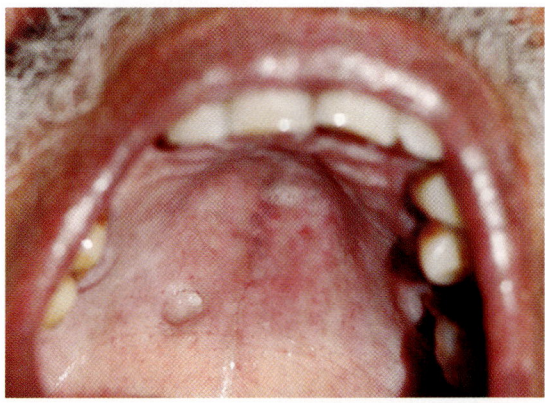

Fig. 5.109: A 49-year-old bidi smoker presented with a pale pink papule on the right to mid-palatine raphae, just anterior to the junction of hard and soft palate. The growth had a well-defined margin, was sessile and firm in consistency.

Papillary Hyperplasia of Palate

It is a reactive inflammatory growth that usually, although not always, develops beneath a denture occurs on hard palate. It may also be seen in bidi smokers. The reported prevalence is 13.9%.

Clinical Presentation

It presents as a cluster of individual papules or nodules which may be erythematous, somewhat translucent or normal in surface coloration. Often the entire vault of the hard palate is involved, with alveolar mucosa being largely spared. There is seldom pain, but a burning sensation may be produced by the yeast infection. Early papules are more edematous while older ones are more fibrotic and firm, being individually indistinguishable from irritation fibroma.

Treatment

For early lesions, removal of dentures and cessation of smoking habit may allow the erythema and edema to subside, and the tissues may resume a more normal appearance. The condition may also show improvement after topical or systemic antifungal therapy.

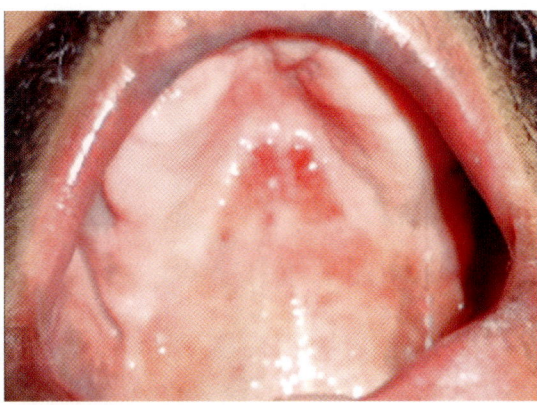

Fig. 5.110: Presence of erythematous papules on the anterior region of palate, on either sides of mid-palatine raphe, in a bidi smoker.

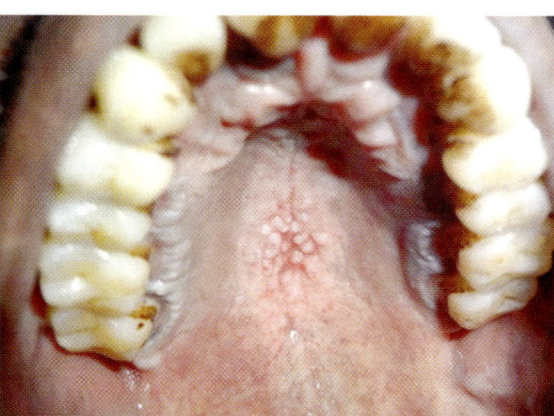

Fig. 5.111: Multiple pale pink papules clustered together associated with nicotinic stomatitis on an erythematous base, in a 43-year-old bidi smoker.

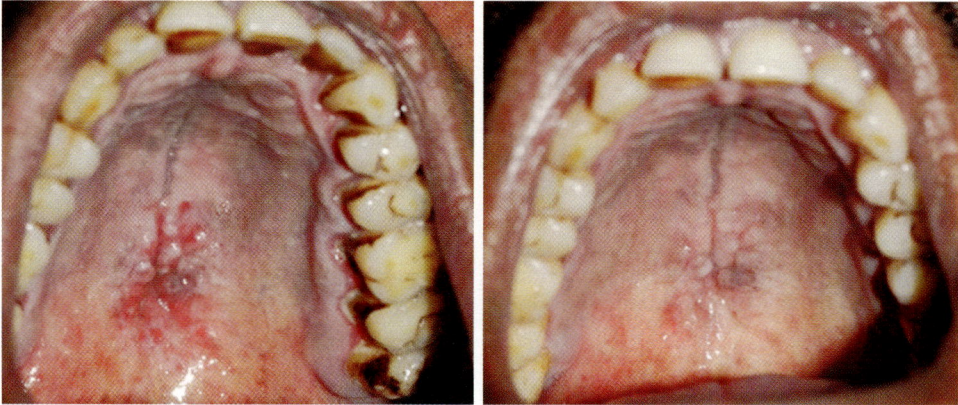

Fig. 5.112: Markedly reduced hyperplasia on application of clotrimazole (Candid mouth paint) for one week.

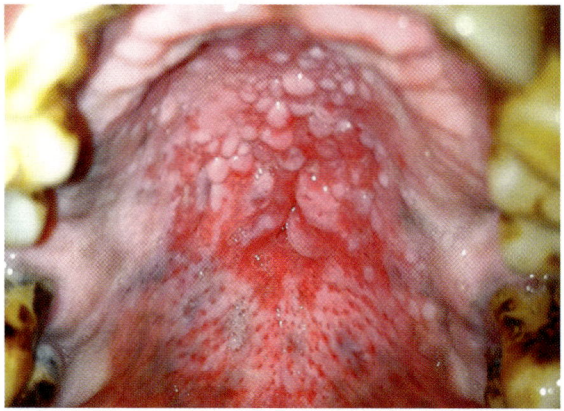

Fig. 5.113: Multiple hyperplastic papules on palate on an erythematous base, in a 51-year-old bidi smoker.

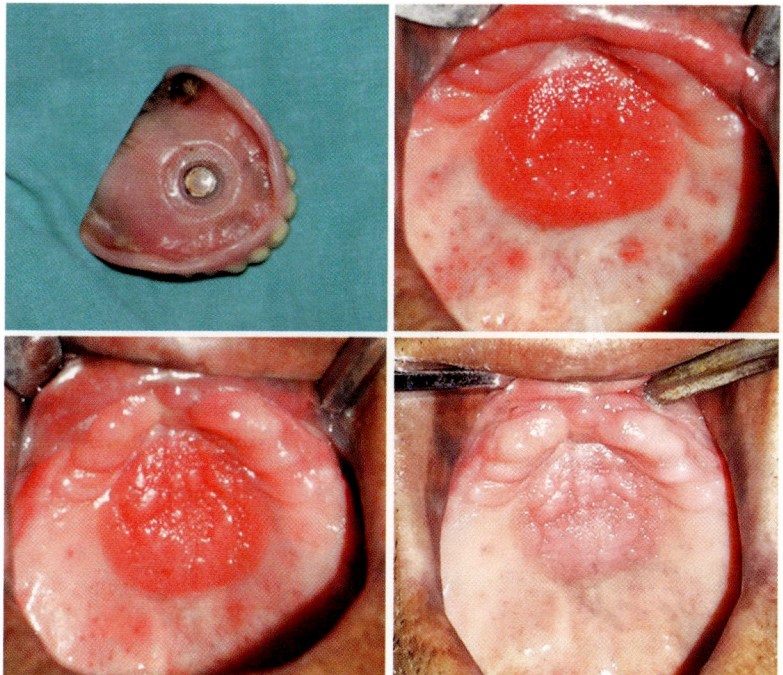

Fig. 5.114: Presence of papillary hyperplasia of palate secondary to complete denture. There is an immense improvement in the erythema and extent of the hyperplastic lesion on palate, on application of clotrimazole (Candid mouth paint).

Erythematous Candidiasis

In several populations, it has been found that about 50% of normal individuals are carriers of Candida. A variety of oral lesions are caused by the fungus *Candida albicans*. The term 'candidiasis' is used when lesions are present. The disease is also known as "moniliasis" and "candidiosis".

Acute candidiasis may be pseudomembranous or atrophic. The former, also known as thrush, consists of creamy-white patches which can be removed by gentle scraping. The atrophic variety, a red painful lesion, may occur during treatment with antibiotics. Chronic candidiasis may manifest in several forms: As persistent angular cheilitis, as denture stomatitis, as a median rhomboid glossitis—like lesion, and as a retrocommissural hyperplastic lesion. The latter may often resemble a leukoplakia.

In erythematous candidiasis, there is a diffused red patch on the palate, which may also be seen in patients other than tobacco users, such as denture wearers and immune-compromised patients.

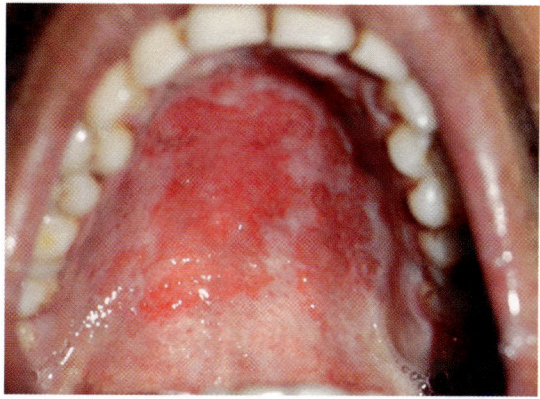

Fig. 5.115: Erythematous candidiasis seen on the palate of a 32-year-old male patient with bidi smoking habit.

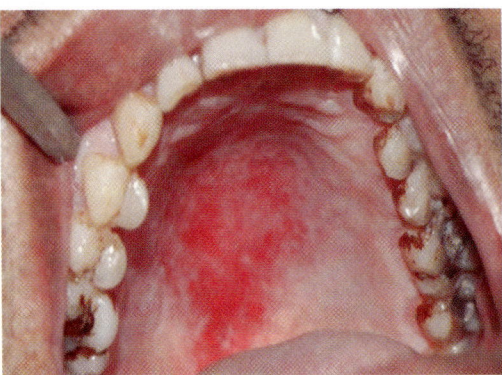

Fig. 5.116: Diffused erythema extending from the posterior extent of rugae to the posterior extent of hard palate, in a 36-year-old bidi smoker.

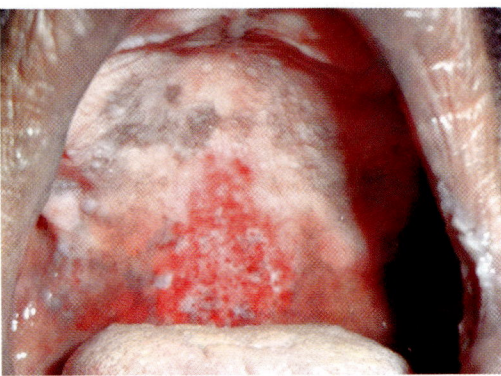

Fig. 5.119: Presence of candidiasis, on the posterior region of hard palate and soft palate, posterior to an area of diffused melanin pigmentation, in a 63-year-old bidi smoker (area of grey discoloration).

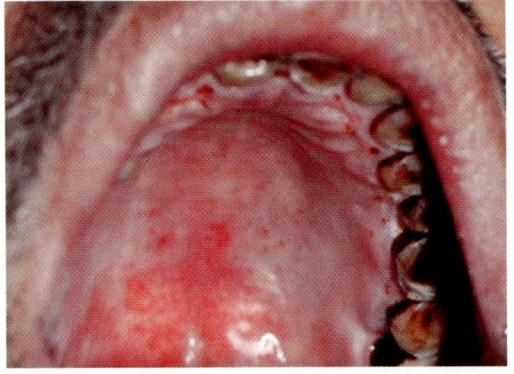

Fig. 5.117: A 40-year-old male with bidi smoking habit presented with a shiny red patch on the posterior region of hard palate.

Nicotinic Stomatitis

Development of greyish mucosa interspersed with pinpoint erythematous areas, representing inflamed ducts of minor salivary glands on the palate in heavy smokers. In the early stages, the mucosa is reddened, but soon becomes greyish-white and may present a wrinkled appearance. Later it becomes thickened and white umbilicated nodules with red centers appear, particularly in the posterior part of the palate. Cancer develops rarely, except in reverse smoker.

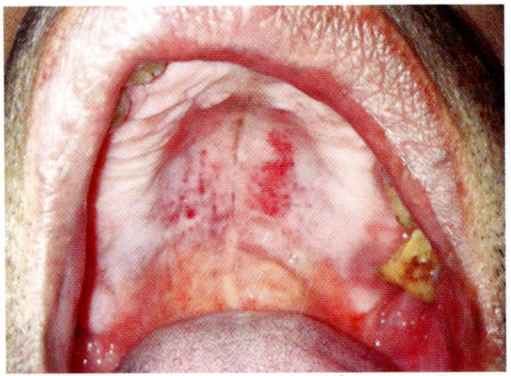

Fig. 5.118: Localized areas of erythema on either sides of mid-palatine raphe, in a 56-year-old denture wearer with bidi smoking habit.

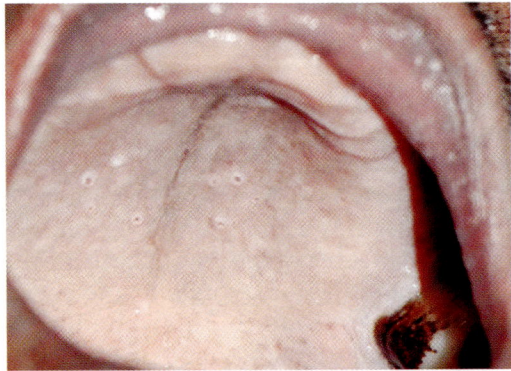

Fig. 5.120: A grey discoloration of the palate with pinpoint erythematous areas, in a 50-year-old bidi smoker.

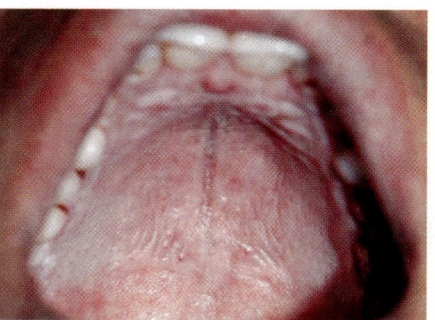

Fig. 5.121: Smoker's palate in a 43-year-old bidi smoker.

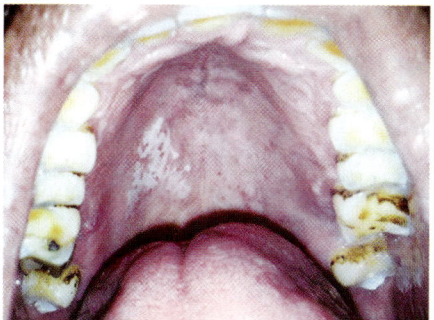

Fig. 5.124: Presence of homogenous leukoplakia on the right side of palate in a 50-year-old bidi smoker.

Verrucous Leukoplakia

Verrucous leukoplakia resembles verrucous carcinoma (Ackerman's tumor). Hansen et al reported a similar form, which was called proliferative verrucous leukoplakia. All areas of oral cavity, including palate, can be affected.

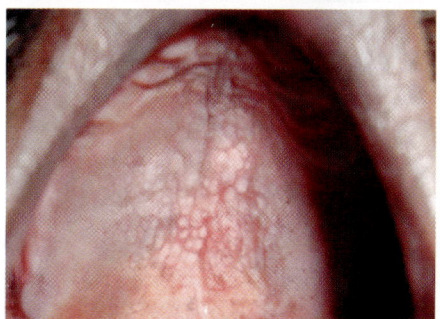

Fig. 5.122: Presence of numerous tiny pale pink papules covering the central portion of hard palate, surrounded by a grey discoloration, in a 57-year-old male with bidi smoking habit.

Pallor

Pallor on the palate may be associated with liver cirrhosis (chronic alcoholism) or anemia or jaundice or oral submucous fibrosis. It can be seen in patients with tobacco habits also. It is important to rule out any underlying cause.

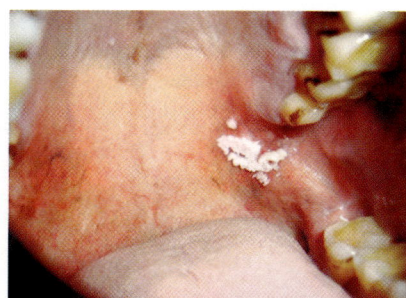

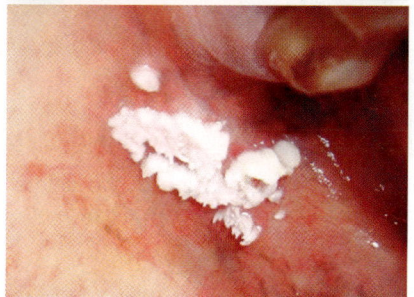

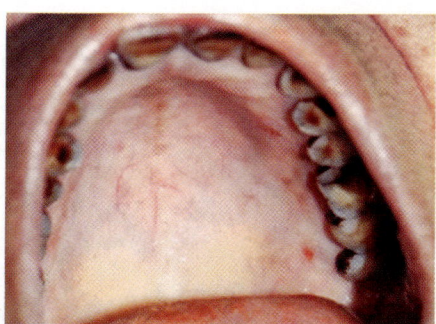

Fig. 5.123: A 52-year-old pan chewer presented with a yellowish color change on the posterior region of palate, suggestive of pallor.

Fig. 5.125: A 55-year-old female presented with localized region of a growth on the left posterior palate region, white in color with numerous finger-like projections, associated with pan chewing habit. An incisional biopsy of the lesion was performed and histopathological features suggested proliferative verrucous leukoplakia.

Oral Submucous Fibrosis

Oral submucous fibrosis will lead to mild to moderate to severe blanching of the palatal mucosa, and decreased mobility of soft tissues of the soft palate, due to increased deposition of fibrous tissue. Patients may complain of difficulty in deglutition. The uvula may appear shrunken or deviated.

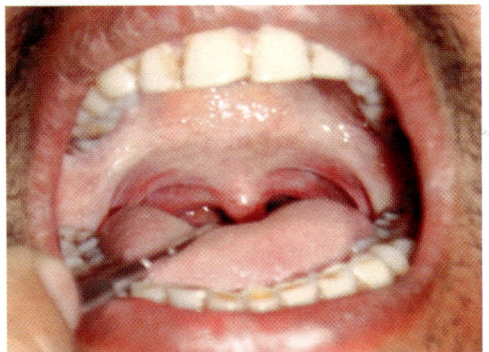

Fig. 5.126: A 32-year-old male with a habit of areca nut chewing presented with blanching of palatal mucosa with a deviated uvula.

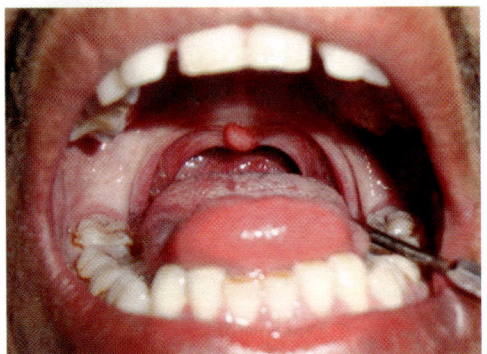

Fig. 5.127: Severe blanching of the palate and a shrunken uvula in a 24-year-old male patient with oral submucous fibrosis.

Carcinoma

Oral cancer may sometimes appear on the palate. Reverse smoking is associated with carcinoma of the palate and posterior part of the dorsum of tongue. The clinical appearance may be an erythematous patch or an ulcerative growth on the palatal mucosa.

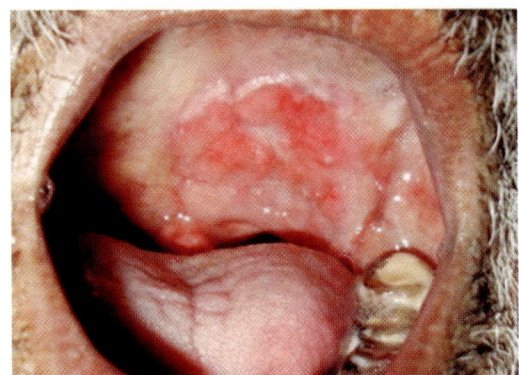

Fig. 5.128: A large, raised patch on the left middle and posterior region of palate, 50-year-old male with bidi smoking habit.

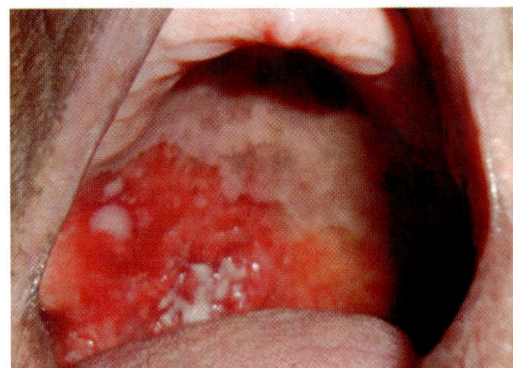

Fig. 5.129: A large erythematous area on the right side of posterior palatal region, interspersed with white nodular specks on the soft palate; in a 59-year-old bidi smoker.

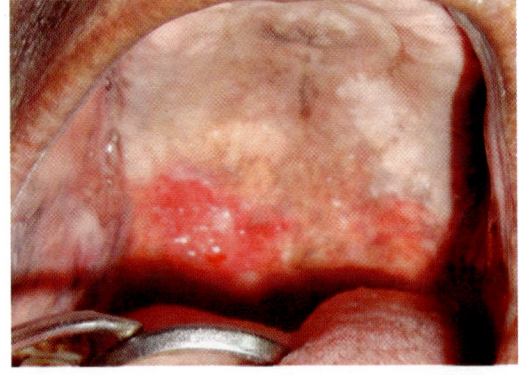

Fig. 5.130: An ill-defined ulcerative lesion present on right half of soft palate with minute papillary projections and bleeding tendency.

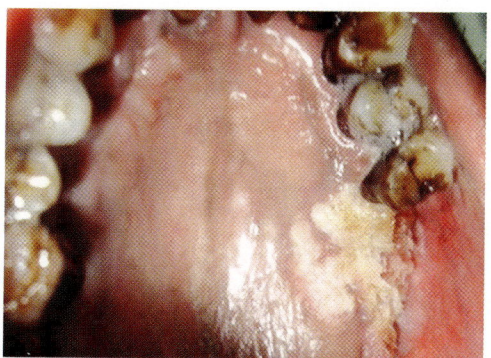

Fig. 5.131: A 52-year-old tobacco chewer presented with a yellowish verrucous growth on the left posterior alveolar ridge and palate, bounded on one side by an erythematous area, with an appearance of burrowing into the alveolar bone; indurated on palpation.

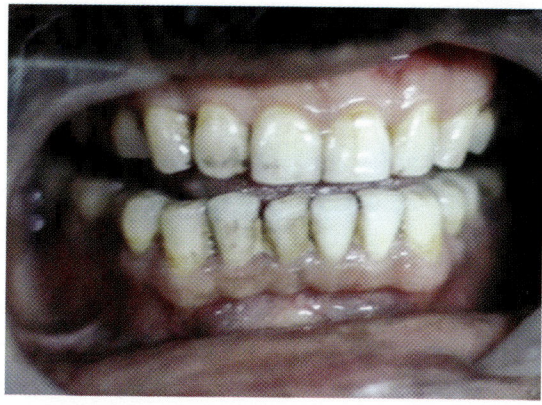

Fig. 5.133: A 45-year-old male with tobacco chewing habit presented with yellow-brown extrinsic stains on teeth.

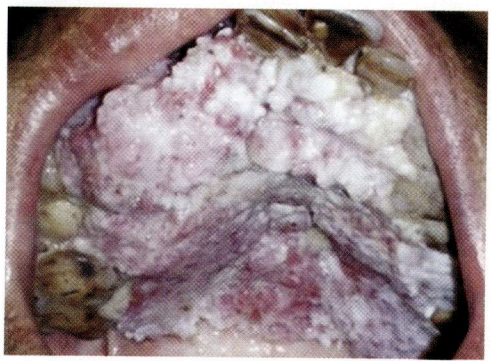

Fig. 5.132: Presence of a widespread verrucous growth on the palate in a 67-year-old female with plain areca nut and pan chewing habits.

EFFECTS OF TOBACCO ON DENTAL TISSUES

Extrinsic Stains on Teeth

Both smoked and smokeless tobacco cause development of extrinsic stains on teeth and exposed parts of roots. There is a significant brown discoloration of the surface enamel. The tar within the tobacco easily dissolves in saliva and penetrates the pits and fissures of enamel. It is most commonly seen on the lingual surfaces of mandibular anterior teeth, in smokers. In smokeless tobacco users, it is seen most commonly at the site of placement of tobacco.

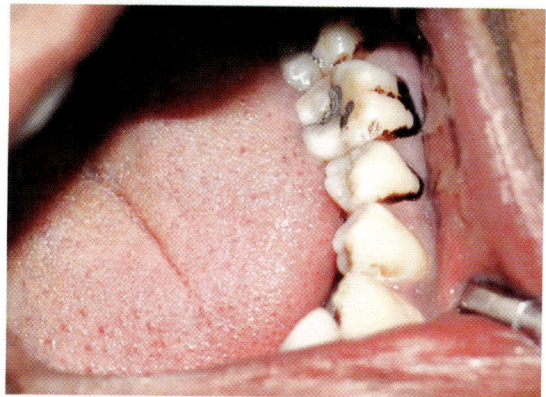

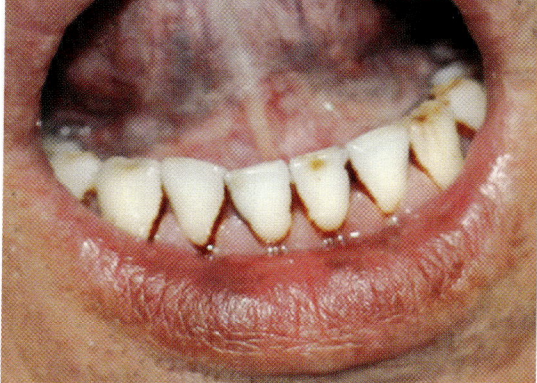

Fig. 5.134: Brown-black extrinsic stains on the cervical region of mandibular anterior and posterior teeth in a 30-year-old male with gutkha and tobacco chewing habit.

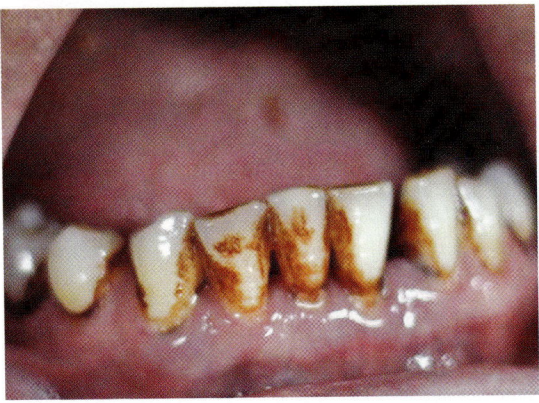

Fig. 5.135: A 35-year-old male presented with gingival recession and periodontal pockets along with brown stains on the labial surface of teeth, associated with pan chewing.

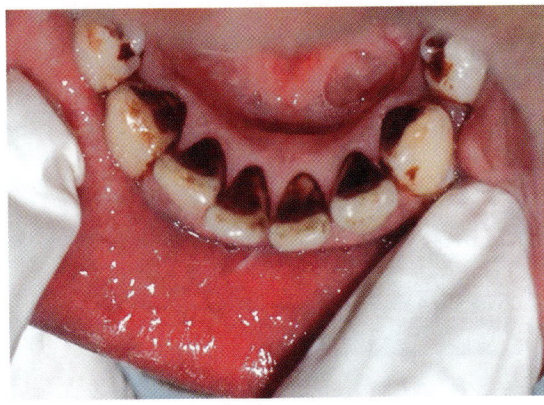

Fig. 5.136: Dark-brown stains covering the entire lingual surfaces of mandibular teeth, in a 25-year-old male with pan chewing habit.

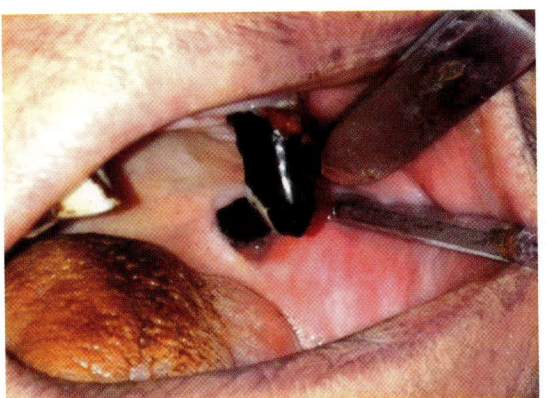

Fig. 5.137: Black discoloration of teeth in a 63-year-old female patient with pan chewing habit.

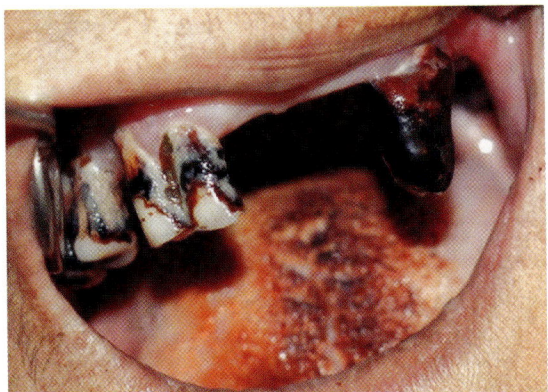

Fig. 5.138: Heavy calculus and stains on teeth in a 62-year-old female patient with pan chewing habit.

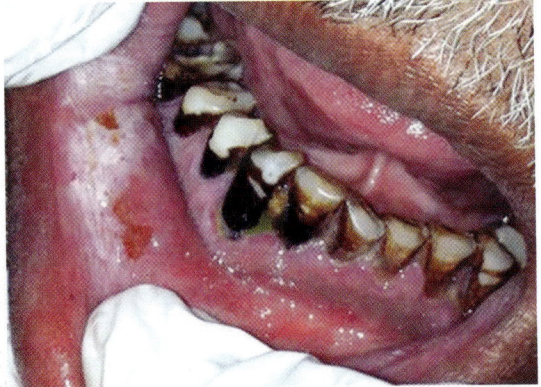

Fig. 5.139: Stains and calculus deposition on mandibular anterior teeth, associated with tobacco and pan chewing habits.

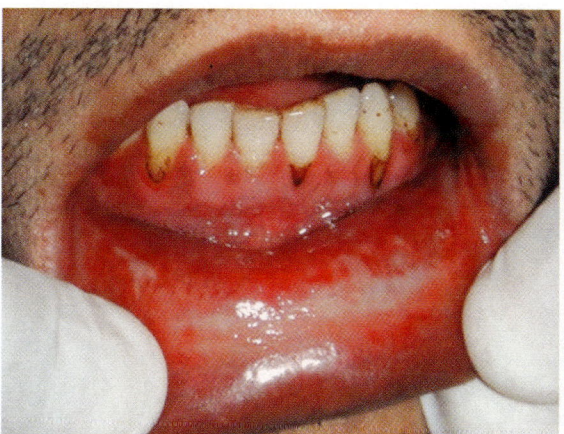

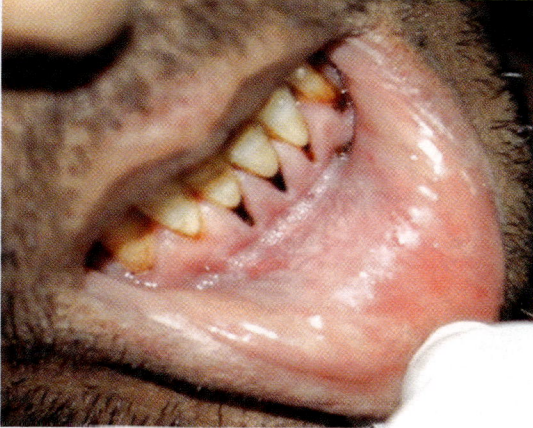

Fig. 5.140: Cervical region exposure and staining due to gingival recession in mandibular anterior teeth, associated with areca nut chewing.

Regressive Changes/Wasting Diseases of Teeth

Tobacco use leads to harmful effects on the hard tissues of oral cavity. Smokeless tobacco use is associated with increased caries (coronal and root) and cervical abrasions. Smokeless tobacco contains a high level of sugar, and is held in one area of the mucosa—typically adjacent to the facial/buccal surfaces of the teeth. In addition, continuous rubbing of teeth with coarse particles of tobacco, causes attrition of teeth. Moreover, already carious teeth become more susceptible to fracture, due to chewing of hard/rough slices of chewable tobacco.

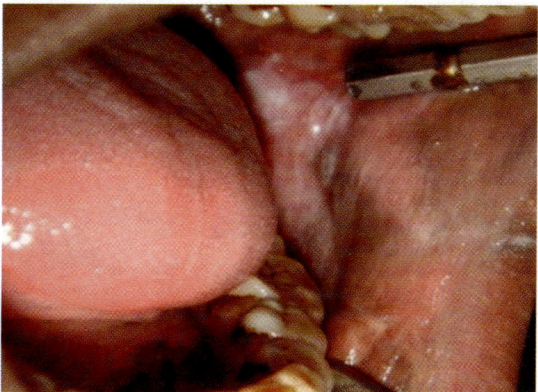

Fig. 5.142: Attrition and stains on teeth associated with bidi smoking on a 50-year-old male patient.

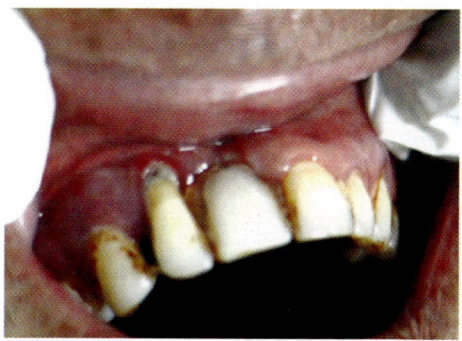

Fig. 5.141: Gingiva recession and cervical abrasion in a 35-year-old male with pan and zarda chewing habits.

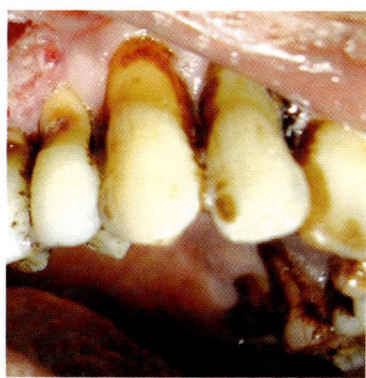

Fig. 5.143: Cervical abrasion (with gingival recession) in a 34-year-old male with tobacco chewing habit.

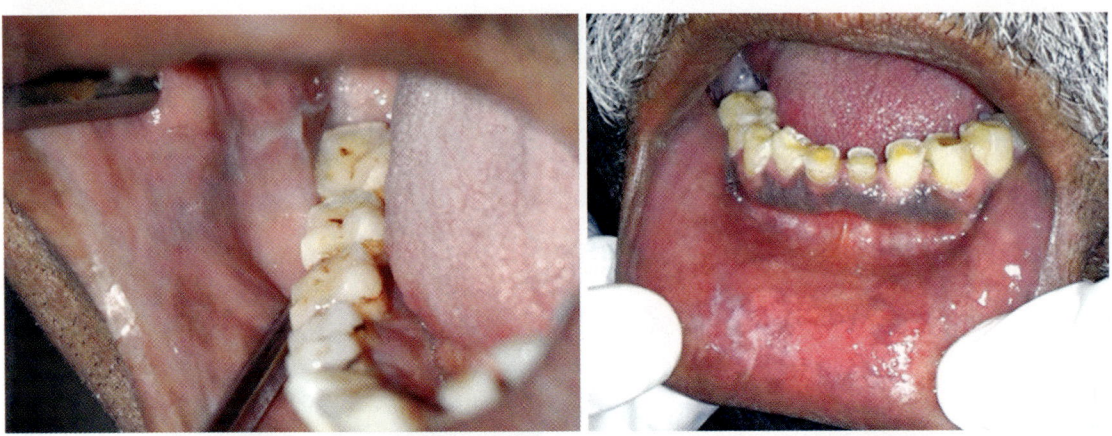

Fig. 5.144: Attrition of teeth, associated with tobacco chewing.

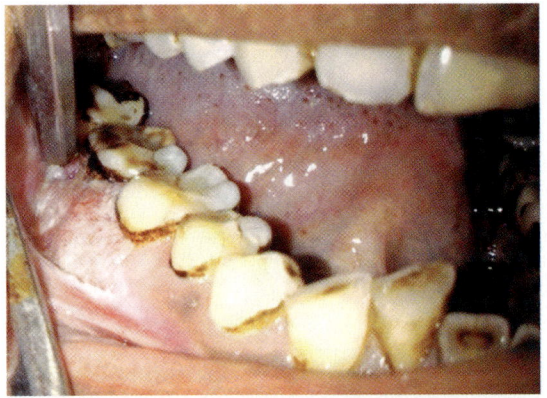

Fig. 5.145: Extrinsic stains and attrited surfaces of mandibular teeth.

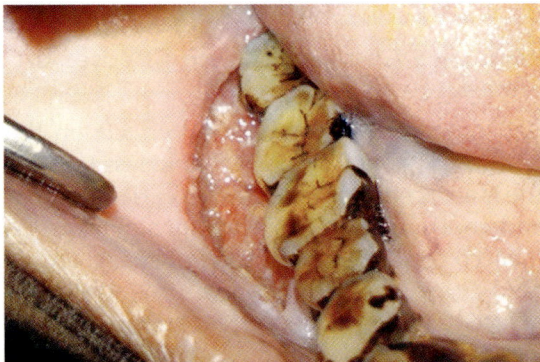

Fig. 5.146: Generalized attrition and dark brown to black colored extrinsic stains in a female patient with tobacco chewing habit.

Tobacco Cessation Centre and Oral Cancer Screening

If we lose the battle against tobacco, we will lose the war against cancer

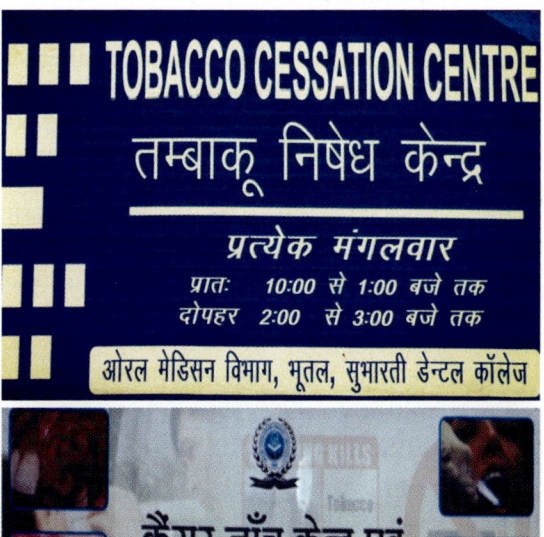

Fig. 6.1: Tobacco Cessation and Oral Cancer Screening Centre (Subharti Dental College and Hospital, Meerut).

> The tobacco companies knew quite early of the addictive nature of their product.
>
> **—Neil Cavuto**

There are approximately 120 million smokers in India. According to the **World Health Organization (WHO),** India is home to 12% of the world's smokers. Approximately 9,00,000 people die every year in India due to smoking as of 2009.

According to a 2002 WHO estimate, 30% of adult males in India smoke. Among adult females, the figure is much lower at between 3 and 5%. These habits are deeply entrenched in the lifestyle of the society, any intervention should go beyond the individual to include family and socio-cultural framework.

Tobacco use is the single most important risk factor in the community and various strategies are being employed for supply reduction and demand reduction of tobacco and its products. The immediate benefits of tobacco control can be seen in those who quit tobacco.

Tobacco Cessation Centres: The Indian Scenario

Tobacco cessation is a relatively new area in tobacco control in India. WHO in collaboration with the government identified **13 tobacco cessation centres** in 2002 in diverse settings (cancer treatment centres, psychiatric centres, medical colleges and NGOs) to help people to stop tobacco use. Most of these clinics were operationalized on the **31st of May, 2002** on the occasion of **World No Tobacco Day.** Tobacco cessation activities formally began with the opening of 13 tobacco cessation clinics in **Anand, Bhopal, Bangalore, Chandigarh, Chennai, Cuttack, Delhi, Goa, Jaipur, Lucknow, Mumbai,** and **Patna** in 2002. Tobacco cessation clinics were renamed to tobacco cessation **centres** in 2005. Five more tobacco cessation centres were established in **Mizoram, Guwahati, Kolkata, Hyderabad** and **Trivandrum,** which makes a total of **18 centres.**

The trained investigators have established centres at various centres and the WHO supports the staff and infrastructure. Each centre has a medical officer, clinical psychologists and medical social workers. Information about the subject is collected on a structured clinical record form. In addition, the software for a standardized patient intake form was developed to ensure uniformity in data collation across the country.

An algorithm was developed which assessed the habit pattern and took the habit through logical approach, initiating with **simple advice, behavioral counselling** and **pharmaceutical treatment.**

The tobacco cessation centres act as foci for community based tobacco control programmes and the centres have undertaken various activities in the community. Corporates have been sensitised and the employees who are habituated to tobacco are being provided with necessary intervention. The centres have also developed health education materials and various posters and pamphlets.

Particularly WHO's **"MPOWER"** policies can counter the tobacco epidemic and reduce its death toll. MPOWER stands for:

1. **M**onitor tobacco use and prevention policies
2. **P**rotect people from tobacco smoke
3. **O**ffer help to quit tobacco use
4. **W**arn about the dangers of tobacco use
5. **E**nforce bans on tobacco advertisements, promotion and sponsorship
6. **R**aise taxes on tobacco

The clinician should bear in mind that quitting tobacco habits can be very difficult, so it is important to be patient and persistent in developing, implementing, and adjusting each patient's tobacco cessation program. One of the most effective behavioral interventions is advice from a health care professional; it seems not to matter whether the advice is from a doctor, respiratory therapist, nurse, or other clinician, so tobacco cessation should be encouraged by multiple clinicians.

Effective tobacco treatment is evidence-based and includes office systems that ensure routine intervention and follow-up. Brief interventions, self-help materials, and **nicotine replacement therapy** for established nicotine dependence form the mainstay of therapy.

The US Public Health Service Guideline recommends that: (a) *all* smokers be offered treatment, (b) patients *unwilling* to quit be provided with a brief intervention to build motivation, and (c) patients *willing* to quit be offered evidence-based treatment. Office-based intervention should follow five major steps (The *"5 As"*) to intervene systematically with patients: *Ask* the patient if she or he uses tobacco; *Advise* him or her to quit; *Assess* willingness to quit; *Assist* with quit attempt; and *Arrange* for follow-up to prevent/address relapse. Model programs in large managed-care organizations suggest that full implementation of the US PHS Guideline increases the use of proven treatments and decreases smoking prevalence.

The **5 Rs** is recommended in the event that tobacco quitting is not being contemplated:

Relevance: Encourage the patient to indicate why quitting is personally relevant, being as specific as possible.

Risks: Dentist can help the patient to identify potential negative consequences of tobacco use. Suggest and highlight those that seem most relevant to the patient.

Rewards: Dentist should ask the patient to identify potential benefits of stopping tobacco use.

Roadblocks: The clinician should ask the patient to identify barriers or impediments to quitting and note elements of treatment.

Repetition: The motivational intervention should be repeated every time an unmotivated patient visits the clinic.

Pharmacotherapy for smoking cessation consists of 7 first-line medications: Bupropion SR, varenicline, and five forms of nicotine replacement therapy (NRT; patch, gum, lozenge, nasal spray, and inhaler). All have been approved for use in treating smoking cessation by the US Food and Drug Administration.

Patients are offered telephonic counseling through **helplines** to be a part of their ongoing battle against tobacco and to virtually follow-up with them. Since, a few patients have a major confidentiality concern, it also aids in concealing the identity and habits of these patients to others and their folks.

Other than all these methods, the following have been tried with success:

a. Audio-visual aids

b. Individual counseling

c. Group counseling

d. Interactive sessions

e. Behavioural modifications

An ideal tobacco cessation program is individualized, accounting for the reasons the person uses tobacco, the environment in which the habit occurs, available resources to quit, and individual preferences about how to quit.

The expansion of tobacco cessation centres is an important part of our historic and continuing effort to help smokers quit. The expansion of these centres will give even more people, the help they need to quit once and for all.

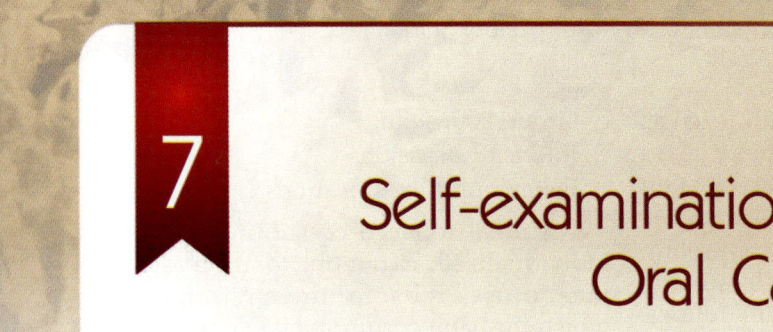

7 Self-examination of Oral Cavity

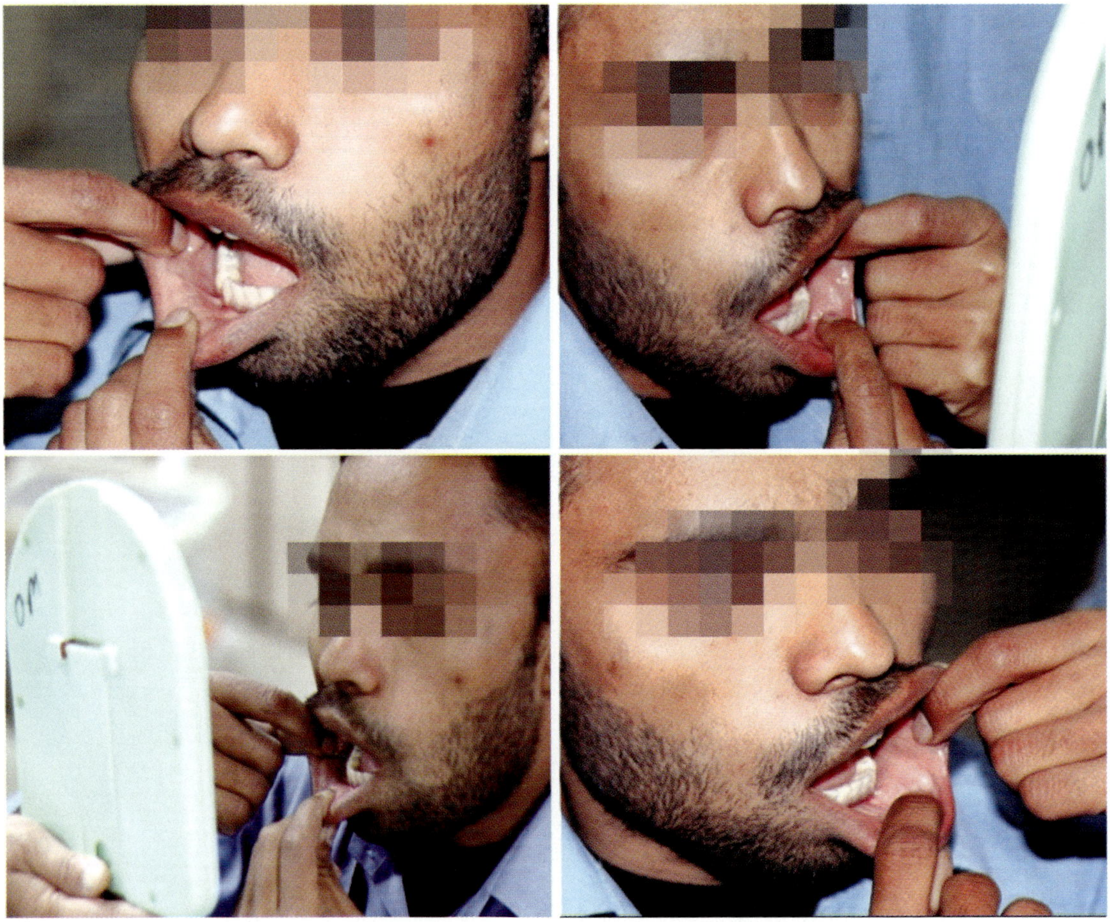

Fig. 7.1: Self-examination of right and left buccal mucosae by a patient.

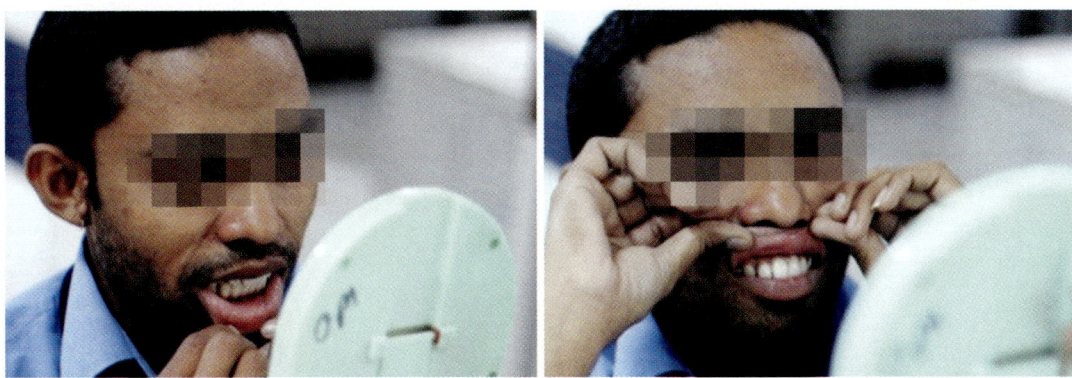

Fig. 7.2: Self-examination of upper and lower labial mucosae respectively by a patient.

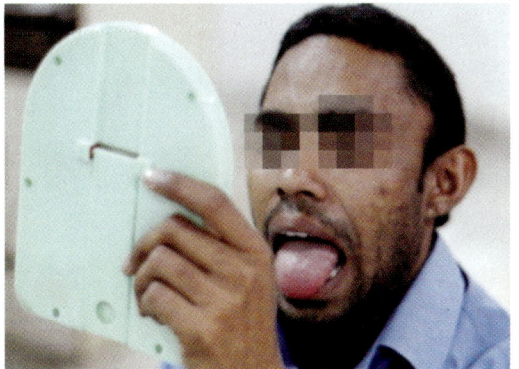

Fig. 7.3: Self-examination of dorsal surface of tongue by a patient.

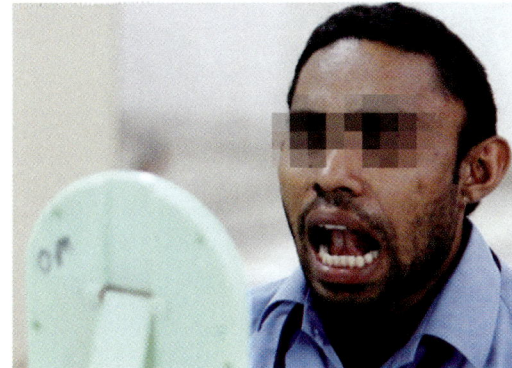

Fig. 7.4: Self-examination of ventral surface of tongue by a patient.

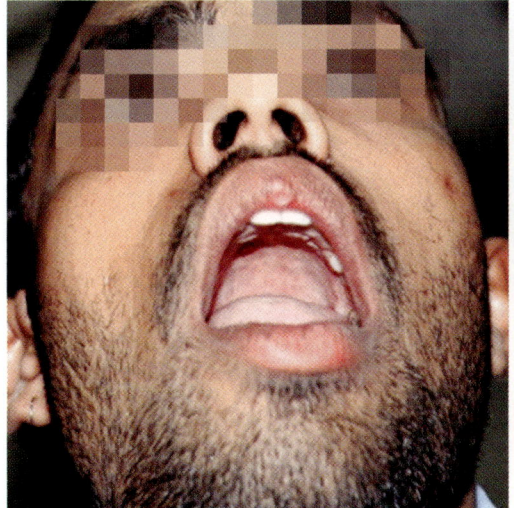

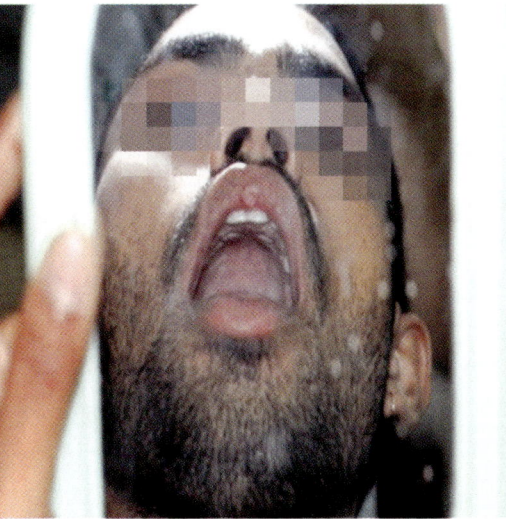

Fig. 7.5: Self-examination of the palate by a patient.

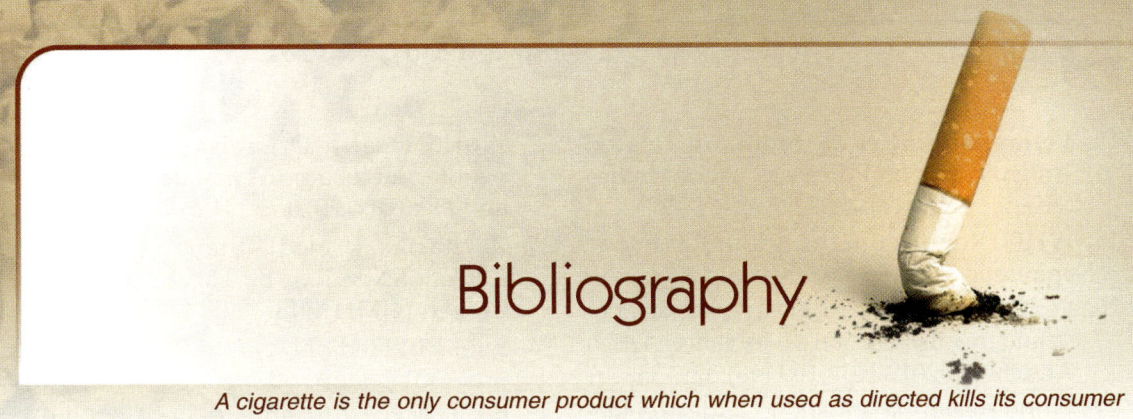

Bibliography

A cigarette is the only consumer product which when used as directed kills its consumer

1. Ajit Auluck, Miriam P. Rosin, Lewei Zhang, Sumanth KN. Oral submucous fibrosis, a clinically benign but potentially malignant disease; Report of 3 Cases and Review of the Literature. JCDA 2008 Oct; 74(8):735–40.

2. Anitha Krishnan P. Fungal infections of the oral mucosa. Indian Journal of Dental Research 2012; 23(5):650–59.

3. M.A.M. Sitheeque and L.P. Samaranayake. Chronic hyperplastic candidosis/candidiasis (Candidal Leukoplakia). Critical Reviews in Oral Biology and Medicine 2003;14(4):253–67.

4. Mehta FS, Hamner JE. Tobacco-related oral mucosal lesions and conditions in India. A guide for Dental Students, Dentists, and Physicians, 1993.

5. Prakash C. Gupta, Samira Asma. Bidi smoking and public health. Ministry of Health and Family Welfare, Government of India World Health Organization.

6. Regezi, et al. Oral pathology. Clinical pathologic correlations, 2008.

7. Reichart PA, Phillipsen HP. Betel chewer's mucosa—a review. J Oral Pathol Med. 1998 Jul; 27(6):239–42.

8. Reichart PA. Philipsen HP. Color Atlas of Dental Medicine, 2000.

9. Report on oral tobacco use and its implications in South-East Asia, WHO Searo, 2004.

10. Richter PK, et al. A rationale and model for addressing tobacco dependence in substance abuse treatment. Substance abuse treatment, prevention, and policy 2006; 1:23.

11. Rogério-Oliveira Gondak, Rogério da Silva-Jorge, Jacks Jorge, Márcio-Ajudarte Lopes, Pablo-Agustin Vargas. Oral pigmented lesions: Clinicopathologic features and review of the literature. Med Oral Patol Oral Cir Bucal 2012 Nov 1;17(6): e919–24.

12. Sigal J.M, Mock D. Symptomatic benign migratory glossitis: Report of two cases and literature review. Pediatr Dent 1992; 14:392–96.

13. Strassburg M, Knolle G. Diseases of the oral mucosa, a color atlas, second edition. Chicago, 1972.

14. Tobacco use in India: An evil with many faces.

15. Tobacco use in India: Practices, patterns and prevalence, p43–47.

16. Trivedy CR, Craig G, Warnakulasuriya S. The oral health consequences of chewing areca nut. Addict Biol 2002 Jan;7(1): 115–25.

17. Varghese C, et al. Initiating tobacco cessation services in India: Challenges and opportunities. WHO South-East Asia Journal of Public Health 2012;1(2): 159–68.

18. Vellappally S, et al. Smoking related systemic and oral diseases. Acta Medica (Hradec Kralove) 2007;50(3):161–66.

19. WHO Report on the global tobacco epidemic, 2008.

20. Wolff KD, Follmann M, Nast A. The diagnosis and treatment of oral cavity cancer. Dtsch Arztebl Int 2012 Nov;109 (48):829–35.

21. World Health Organisation. Guide to epidemiology and diagnosis of oral mucosal diseases and conditions. Munksgaard, Copenhagen, 1980.

22. World Health Organisation. Helping people quit tobacco. A manual for Doctors and Dentists, 2010.

23. Zacharias J. et al. Starting Tobacco Cessation Services, by Tobacco Cessation Center, NIMHANS.

24. Zain RB, Ikeda N, Gupta PC, et al. Oral mucosal lesions associated with betel quid, areca nut and tobacco chewing habits: Consensus from a workshop held in Kuala Lumpur, Malaysia; J Oral Pathol Med 1996;28:1–4.

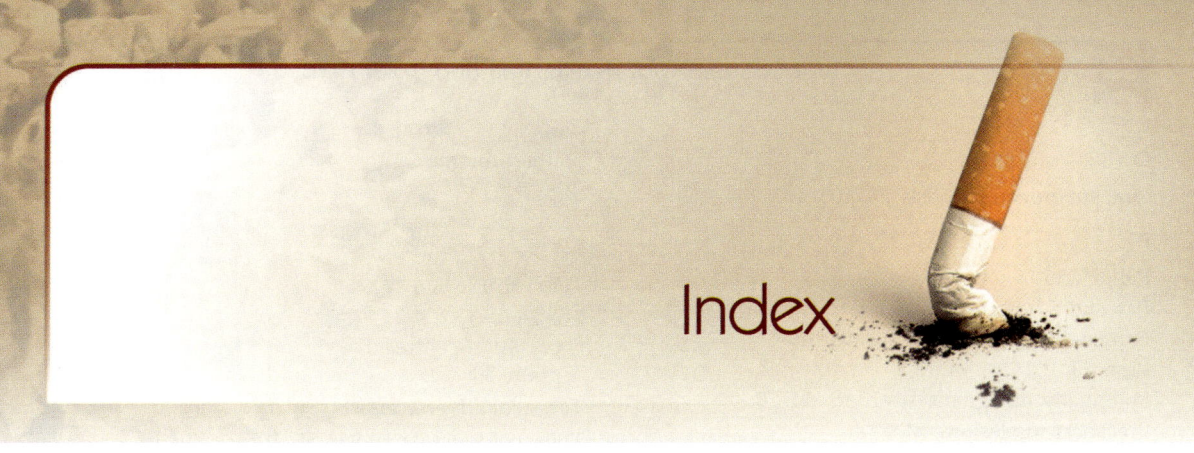

Index